Telephone Triage Care

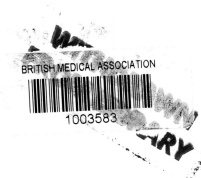

Telephone Triage Care

Edited by Claire Hunter

CLASS PROFESSIONAL PUBLISHING

Disclaimer

Class Professional Publishing and its contributors (including NHS Digital), (collectively 'the Suppliers' or 'We' or 'Our' as the context admits) have taken steps to ensure that the information, tables, drawings and diagrams contained in this book are accurate at the time of publication. Users of this book ('You'/'Your') must always be aware that innovations or alterations in medical or procedural practice after the date of publication may not be incorporated in the content and use of this book is not intended to be a substitute for suitable training and/or consultation with a suitable health professional. You hereby agree that this book cannot always contain all the information necessary for determining appropriate care and cannot address all individual situations; therefore, You and all individuals You permit to use the book must ensure You and they have the appropriate knowledge and skills to enable suitable interpretation.

The Suppliers shall not be liable and shall not compensate You or any other party for any loss or damage You may suffer unless we have breached any duties imposed on us by law, including if We have caused death or personal injury by Our negligence and that failure is not attributed to: (a) Your own fault; (b) the fault of a third party; or (c) any other events which We could not have foreseen or forestalled even if We had taken reasonable care.

Please note, however, the Suppliers assume no responsibility whatsoever for the content of external resources referred to in the text or accompanying online materials.

This first edition published 2018

The publishers and authors welcome feedback from readers of this edition.

Class Professional Publishing
The Exchange, Express Park, Bristol Road, Bridgwater TA6 4RR
Email: editorial@class.co.uk
www.classprofessional.co.uk
Class Professional Publishing is an imprint of Class Publishing Ltd
A CIP catalogue record for this book is available from the British Library
ISBN 9781859597859 (paperback)
ISBN 9781859597866 (ebook)

Cover design by Hybert Design Limited, UK
Designed and typeset by RefineCatch Limited, Bungay, Suffolk
Printed in the UK by Bell & Bain Limited

Contents

Contributors

Claire Hunter, Bachelor of Nursing (Hons), RGN, PGCE, works for NHS Digital as the national Head of Learning, Development and Quality for NHS Pathways, a post she has held since 2004. Claire, a nurse by background, has extensive experience within the field of telephone triage. She previously worked for NHS Direct both in a clinical capacity and as the North West Head of Education. Claire also has experience within community nursing and public health. She is a strong advocate for the call handling role within telephone triage, believing that with high-quality education and training, call handlers can carry out this complex role safely and effectively. A staunch believer in the importance of promoting healthy and happy workplaces, Claire is also a mindfulness instructor, life coach and Mental Health First Aid instructor.

Andy Inniss, DipM, BA (Hons), Cert. Ed., HND, lives in the West Country and works for South Western Ambulance Service NHS Foundation Trust within the 999 Clinical Hub Education Team. He joined the NHS ambulance service in 1999 and has worked in training roles since 2004. This has included working as an accredited instructor for Criteria Based Dispatch, National Instructor (Advanced Medical Priority Dispatch System) and as an accredited NHS Pathways instructor (999 & 111). Key project work includes the introduction of two emergency medical telephone triage systems, new computer-aided dispatch systems and an integrated communications control system. During this time, he has also worked as an associate lecturer at Plymouth University, spent five years as a community first responder and became a member of the national trailblazer group comprising police, fire, ambulance and urgent care services developing the Emergency Services Contact Handler apprenticeship.

Sarah Crichton, BA (Hons), Cert. Ed., lives in Northumberland and works for North East Ambulance Service (NEAS) NHS Foundation Trust as the Training Lead for the Operations Centre. She has 21 years of experience in the Operations Centre. Her roles within NEAS have included 999 and out-of-hours call handler, working in dispatch, Criteria Based Dispatch (CBD) Instructor and an accredited NHS Pathways trainer. Key project work includes the introduction of a new computer-aided dispatch system, new radio systems and change of triage systems as well as the introduction of the 111 call handling service in the North East. She is also a member of the NHS Pathways 999 user group and NHS Pathways Training Stakeholder group.

Runveer Dhaliwal, Adult RGN, works for London Central & West Unscheduled Care Collaborative as the Training and Development Manager. She has experience in telephone triage since 2013 which includes using a clinical decision support system, auditing and training. She has developed training sessions as well as guides for telephone triage which are used internally. Runveer has clinical experience in gynaecology, general surgery, orthopaedics and long-term conditions. Runveer has also been trained in colon hydrotherapy, first aid instruction and hypnotherapy as well as in facial aesthetics and learning and education.

Richard Berry, City & Guilds Level 4 Certificate in Education and Training. Richard works for NHS Pathways as an Organisational Development and Learning Officer and has held this post since May 2014. Prior to this he was based at the 111 service in West London as Regional Training Manager where, as part of the senior management team, he supported the implementation of the first live 111 service in London. Richard has worked in the health industry for 17 years, and has extensive experience of telephone triage and the call centre environment. He has been involved in the learning and development field since joining NHS Direct, Hampshire in 2000. Richard has a passion for mental health and sits on the NHS England 111 Mental Health Board. In his spare time he is a Samaritan volunteer and trainer in a Berkshire branch of the charity. He is a qualified Mental Health First Aider in the workplace and is about to train as a Mental Health First Aid Instructor. He believes in talking openly and honestly about the issues that surround mental health in order to break down stigma and taboo.

Sarah Jackson qualified in 2004 as a learning disability nurse and completed an MSc in Advanced Practice specialising in autism and physical health in 2011. Sarah has worked in a variety of inpatient and community settings with people with learning disabilities, autism or both. Her current role is within NHS England's Learning Disability programme as an Associate Clinical Lead for Autism.

Katy Lockhart, BSc (Hons) Biomedical Science, HCPC Paramedic, PGCert. Practice Development, has worked for NHS Digital as a clinical trainer and most recently a clinical systems developer for NHS Pathways. Katy, a paramedic by background, began her career with the North East Ambulance Service and has undertaken the role of paramedic mentor and clinical supervisor within the 999 and 111 settings. She is passionate about establishing effective clinical support for the call handling role within telephone triage and believes that this can be achieved through exceptional training and development of the workforce.

Karen Murray supports self-advocacy groups across North Yorkshire for KeyRing Living Support Networks to encourage people with a learning disability to speak out about things that are important to them. Karen is also a Trustee for Ripon Community Link and writes stories and poems for and about young people and adults with a learning disability.

Carl Shaw has a mild learning disability and previously worked for Dimensions, a national voluntary sector organisation that provides community services for people with learning disabilities and autism for over eight years as a Quality Auditor which involved visiting people in their home to see if they were getting good quality services and living the life they choose. His current role is within NHS England's national Transforming Care and Learning Disability programme. As part of his role Carl has been responsible for carrying out Care and Treatment Reviews for people with learning disabilities, autism or both. He has also co-lead on a project called STOMP which stands for Stop Over Medicating People with learning disabilities, autism or both and is about stopping people being wrongly prescribed psychotropic medication as well as being overmedicated. It supports people in getting the right care, support and treatment. Carl now co-leads on a piece of work with Sarah Jackson called Ask Listen Do which supports people with learning disabilities and autism, in giving feedback, raising concerns and making complaints.

Acknowledgements

The authors and Class Professional Publishing would like to thank the following for their invaluable feedback on this text during its development:

- Sian Ashford
- Deborah Bilton
- David Davis
- Jamie Foster
- Tendai Mhizha
- Manika Power
- Luci Stephens
- Chris Wiseman

Material in chapters 5, 6, 8 and 9 has been reproduced from: Richard Pilbery and Kris Lethbridge, *Ambulance Care Practice*, Bridgwater: Class Publishing (2016), with kind permission from the authors.

With special thanks also to Jane Brooker for her helpful feedback and input on the text.
We would like to thank and acknowledge SWASFT for providing photographs.

Introduction

This textbook is designed to help prepare and support you for a call handling role within the ambulance service, NHS 111 or any other health-based telephone triage service in England. The content is designed for call handlers without a formal clinical qualification.

The book has been designed to complement the training that you will receive to prepare you for your role, irrespective of any differences in the tools, processes and working practices used within your organisation.

Each chapter comprises a number of topics focusing on a common theme. For example, the chapter on telephone communication includes topics such as active listening, negotiation skills and skilled questioning.

The chapters are designed to be read sequentially because concepts introduced later on in the book assume that you already have knowledge of the content covered earlier. Once you have read each chapter, however, it is anticipated that the book will form an invaluable reference tool which can be dipped into and referred to again and again.

There are a number of 'time out activities' within each chapter. It is advisable that you obtain a journal or notebook to record your work on these activities. These activities have been included to help bring the content alive and to actively engage you in thinking about the content of the book.

Each chapter is split into sections, which are typically laid out in the following way:

- Learning objectives: to clearly highlight what you are expected to learn in the chapter.
- Introduction: setting the scene for the theme of the chapter.
- Content: the main body of information relating to the subject.
- Summary: to summarise the key points covered.

Chapter 1: The Healthcare System

Learning Objectives

By the end of this chapter you will be able to:

- Describe the core principles and priorities of the NHS
- Identify the broad structure of the NHS and organisations associated with it
- Distinguish between primary and secondary care
- List the regulators involved in providing telephone triage within the UK
- Discuss NHS funding and modern day pressures on the service
- Present a balanced view of the public's perception of the NHS.

Introduction

The NHS was founded in 1948 by health secretary Aneurin Bevan to establish a good standard of healthcare, which was available to all, irrespective of wealth. New treatments for an increasing and ageing population mean that pressures on the service are greater than ever before. Nevertheless, treatment outcomes are far better and public satisfaction is higher than ten or twenty years ago [DoH, 2017].

The NHS Constitution, first published in 2009, is a framework which summarises the ethos of the NHS and the responsibilities it has to staff and patients. An overview of this framework is set out here:

1. The NHS provides a comprehensive service, available to all.
2. Access to NHS services is based on clinical need, not ability to pay.
3. The NHS aspires to the highest standards of excellence and professionalism.
4. The patient will be at the heart of everything the NHS does.
5. The NHS works across organisational boundaries.
6. The NHS is committed to providing best value for taxpayers' money.
7. The NHS is accountable to the public, communities and patients that it serves.

[DoH, 2015]

With the exception of some charges such as dental care, prescriptions and optical services, the NHS in England remains free to all UK residents. It manages over 1 million patients every 36 hours and provides care across the whole lifespan, including antenatal care, emergency and urgent care, routine screenings such as cervical smear testing, treatments for chronic and life limiting conditions, transplants and end-of-life care [DoH, 2017].

The Structure of the NHS

The NHS is a complex system which is always changing. However, for anyone involved in the delivery of NHS care, it can be really useful to have an overview of some of the main structures.

- **The Secretary of State for Health** is a UK government position. This individual is responsible for the Department of Health, ensuring that the NHS performs effectively and delivers high-quality care.
- **The Department of Health (DoH)** is the parliamentary department responsible for delivering health and social care in England.
- **Public Health England** is part of the DoH. Its mission is 'to protect and improve the nation's health and to address inequalities' [Public Health England, 2017] by advising and supporting the government.
- **NHS England** is an independent body that works alongside the government to set the direction and priorities of the NHS so that improvements can be made in health and care outcomes [NHS, 2017a].
- **Clinical Commissioning Groups (CCGs)** replaced primary care trusts in 2013 following major changes to the structure of health services in England. CCGs are GP-led NHS organisations that organise and commission or 'buy' healthcare such as urgent and emergency

care and mental health services for their local area [NHS Clinical Commissioners, 2017].

- **Vanguards** were set up in 2015 as part of the NHS Five-Year Forward View. Fifty vanguard sites were chosen to lead on developing ways of delivering services [NHS, 2017b].

Care Providers within the NHS

There are various providers of care in the NHS. The two main categories are primary and secondary care.

Primary care is generally the first point of contact for healthcare for most people and around 90% of patient interaction is with primary care services. General practice provides over 300 million patient consultations each year, compared to 23 million emergency department visits [DoH, 2017]. Primary care services are provided by GPs, district nurses, specialist nurses, pharmacists, optometrists, dentists plus other professionals such as physiotherapists and occupational therapists, as well as minor injury units, walk-in centres and the NHS 111 telephone service.

The aim of primary care is to enable easy access to suitable care, whatever the patient's problem, and primary care is the front door to many other parts of the NHS. Primary healthcare is based on caring for people rather than specific diseases. This means that many professionals working in primary care are generalists, dealing with a broad range of physical, psychological and social problems, rather than specialists in any particular disease area.

An important role for primary care is acting as the patient's 'advocate' and coordinating the care of patients with multiple or complex health problems. Primary care practitioners often provide long-term care for patients and the relationships between patient and professional can be particularly important. Primary healthcare involves providing treatment for common illnesses, the management of long-term illnesses such as diabetes and heart disease and the prevention of future ill health through advice, immunisation and screening programmes. A significant amount of minor surgery also takes place within a primary care setting.

Secondary care services are usually (but not always) located in a hospital or clinic and are commissioned by local CCGs. A patient who has been provided with primary care may be referred to a secondary care professional – a specialist with expertise on the patient's issue.

Emergency Care Services

Emergency care services such as the ambulance service and emergency departments have a primary role of supporting patients with immediate medical need, for example serious accidents and serious medical conditions including heart attacks and strokes.

Regulation of NHS Services

Regulation or safeguarding of NHS services is vital and certain organisations are responsible for overseeing this in the NHS.

The Care Quality Commission (CQC) is responsible for monitoring, inspecting and regulating health and care services to ensure they meet essential quality and safety standards [Care Quality Commission, 2016].

Monitor, which operates under the umbrella of NHS Improvements, is the financial regulator. It holds NHS foundation trusts accountable by authorising, monitoring and regulating services to ensure they deliver safe and high-quality care that is economically sustainable [Monitor, 2017].

Healthwatch is an organisation which champions patient views in healthcare in England.

Professional regulatory bodies, such as the General Medical Council, Nursing and Midwifery Council and Health and Care Professions Council, protect the public by providing professional standards and codes of conduct that registered healthcare professionals must adhere to.

Other Structures Relating to the NHS

There are many other supporting organisations that contribute to the NHS.

- **Health Education England** supports the NHS by ensuring its workforce has the appropriate competencies to be able to deliver safe, high-quality care.

- **The National Institute of Health and Care Excellence (NICE)** provides national evidence-based guidance and advice to healthcare professionals to promote the delivery of care that is based on sound evidence and research.

- **NHS Digital**, formerly known as the Health and Social Care Information Centre, plays a vital role in the NHS by providing technology and information. It provides technology such as NHS Pathways that supports the triage of urgent and emergency calls. Information and data provided by NHS Digital enables the audit and analysis of care and outcomes of the NHS. This organisation also provides the 'Spine' which stores demographic information about each patient and their NHS number allowing information to be shared securely [DoH, 2013].

Figure 1.1 is taken from 'Guide to the Healthcare System in England'. It is a useful representation of how some of the organisations discussed here fit together.

NHS Funding, Pressures and Public Perception

The NHS is funded mainly by taxation with a small proportion gained from National Insurance contributions and patient charges such as dental care, prescriptions and optical care [King's Fund, 2017a]. Understandably, spending in the NHS has increased dramatically since it was founded in 1948 and today's budget sits at about £120 billion per year. It is probably not news to you that the NHS faces considerable financial challenges, due in large part to our ever-increasing ageing population. It costs around three times more to look after a 75-year-old than a 30-year-old and today there are half a million more people aged over 75 than there were in 2010 [DoH, 2017].

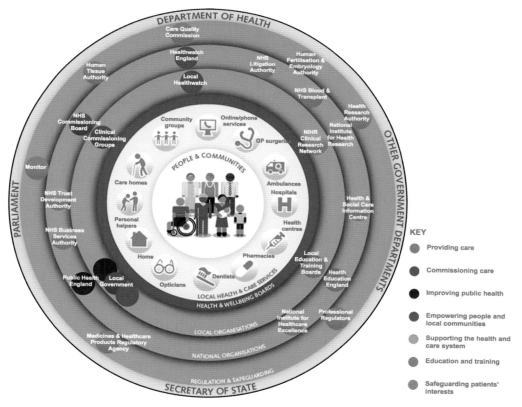

Figure 1.1 Guide to the Healthcare System in England
Source: DoH (2013)

Pressures on the NHS are greater than they have ever been. We are getting healthier but using the NHS more. Demand is also heavily impacted by rising public expectations for convenient and personal care [DoH, 2017].

Research shows that the public are highly satisfied with the NHS, but concerned for its future. Interestingly, 69% of the public in this country say they experience good healthcare compared with 57% in France and 59% in Germany, but a higher proportion of our public are worried about the future of the NHS [King's Fund, 2017b]. In 2014, the Commonwealth Fund reported that in comparison with the healthcare systems of ten other nations (Australia, Canada, France, Germany, Netherlands, New Zealand, Norway, Sweden, Switzerland and the US) the NHS rated as the best in terms of quality and coordination of care, efficiency, patient-centred care and cost-related factors [NHS Choices, 2015].

Summary

The National Health Service is an incredibly complex and ever-changing system of inter-locking organisations. It is not possible or even necessary to know everything there is to know about the NHS and how it works. However, having a basic understanding of certain fundamentals such as the principles, structure, funding and pressures facing the service can help you feel more confident and competent in your important role of delivering care on behalf of the NHS.

The NHS is subject to a significant amount of bad press, but it is worth remembering that there is high public satisfaction with the service and that it compares very favourably with other healthcare systems across the globe. You have an important role to play in ensuring that the public receive the safe and effective care they deserve, and that you deliver this care in a way which recognises the enormous pressures facing the NHS.

References and Further Reading

Care Quality Commission (2016). *Who We Are*. Available at: www.cqc.org.uk/content/who-we-are (last accessed 23 March 2017).

Department of Health (2013). *Guide to the Healthcare System in England*. Available at: www.gov.uk/government/uploads/system/uploads/attachment_data/file/194002/9421-2900878-TSO-NHS_Guide_to_Healthcare_WEB.PDF (last accessed 14 March 2017).

Department of Health (2015). *The NHS Constitution: The NHS Belongs to Us All*. Available at: www.gov.uk/government/uploads/system/uploads/attachment_data/file/480482/NHS_Constitution_WEB.pdf (last accessed 24 March 2017).

Department of Health (2017). *Next Steps on the NHS Five-Year Forward View*. Available at: www.england.nhs.uk/wp-content/uploads/2017/03/NEXT-STEPS-ON-THE-NHS-FIVE-YEAR-FORWARD-VIEW.pdf (last accessed 19 April 2017).

King's Fund (2017a). *How the NHS is Funded*. [Online]. Available at: www.kingsfund.org.uk/projects/nhs-in-a-nutshell/how-nhs-funded (last accessed 23 March 2017).

King's Fund (2017b). *Public Satisfaction with the NHS and Social Care in 2017*. Available at: https://www.kingsfund.org.uk/publications/public-satisfaction-nhs-2017 (last accessed 4 June 2018).

Monitor (2017). *About Us*. Available at: www.gov.uk/government/organisations/monitor/about (last accessed 24 March 2017).

NHS Choices (2015). *About the NHS*. Available at: www.nhs.uk/NHSEngland/thenhs/about/Pages/nhscoreprinciples.aspx (last accessed 14 March 2017).

NHS Clinical Commissioners (2017). *About CCGs*. Available at: www.nhscc.org/ccgs/ (last accessed 23 March 2017).

NHS England (2017a). *About NHS England*. Available at: https://www.england.nhs.uk/about/about-nhs-england/ (last accessed 24 March 2017).

NHS England (2017b). *About Vanguards*. Available at: www.england.nhs.uk/ourwork/new-care-models/vanguards/about-vanguards/ (last accessed 22 March 2017).

Pilbery, R. and Lethbridge, K. (2016). *Ambulance Care Practice*. Bridgwater: Class Publishing.

Public Health England (2017). *About Us*. Available at: www.gov.uk/government/organisations/public-health-england/about (last accessed 22 March 2017).

Chapter 2: Understanding Telephone Triage and Your Role Within It

Learning Objectives

By the end of this chapter you will be able to:

- Describe telephone triage
- Explain the need for telephone triage
- List examples of who/what is affected by the outcomes of telephone triage
- Describe the complexity of telephone triage
- Discuss the role of clinical decision support systems
- Explain the limits of telephone triage
- Outline the role and boundaries of the call handling role
- Discuss call patterns to telephone triage services.

What is Telephone Triage?

The concept of triage is not new and the practice was first developed on the battlefields by Napoleon's surgeon-general, as a way of deciding the priority with which to help casualties with different forms and severity of injury. The word 'triage' comes from the French verb 'trier', which means 'to sort'.

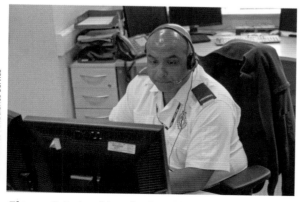

Figure 2.1 A call handler in a 999 control room

Telephone triage is used in many countries across the world today, but the UK has some of the largest and most sophisticated telephone triage services in the world. The aim of modern-day telephone triage within the UK is not to diagnose, but to improve access to healthcare, and to direct patients to the best form of care for their needs.

Why Do We Triage?

In a perfect world, we would have no need to triage anyone, as everyone would have quick and easy access to the medical skill and resources they need. However, we do not live in such a world; it is a feature of today's NHS that demand for services is outstripping supply. Therefore, it is vital that all healthcare staff carry out their roles as efficiently as possible to deliver services to as many patients in need as possible.

Let's consider an illustration of this, using the ambulance service as an example. It could be argued that sending an ambulance to a person with a broken leg is more appropriate than referring them to their local doctor, as the patient clearly needs the services of an emergency department. However, there are likely to be patients who have an even more pressing need for an ambulance, such as someone having a heart attack or a child that has stopped breathing.

Telephone triage enables such needs to be prioritised so that precious and finite health service resources can be used appropriately. Making sure that patients receive the right care, at the right time, in the right clinical environment is important for patients and services.

Competent telephone triage contributes to a positive healthcare cycle. Conversely, a poor triage outcome plays a part in perpetuating a negative cycle of healthcare. These processes are explained in Figures 2.2 and 2.3.

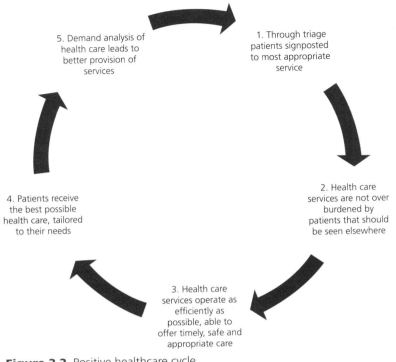

Figure 2.2 Positive healthcare cycle

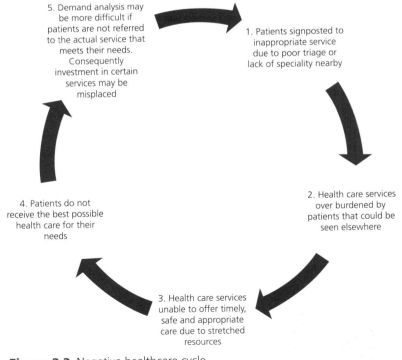

Figure 2.3 Negative healthcare cycle

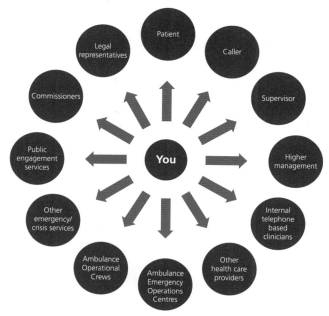

Figure 2.4 Your role in the healthcare system

Who is Affected by the Work You Do?

The healthcare system is a complex set of inter-related systems and it is important to realise that what you do in your role has a significant impact both on the patient and on other parts of the system. Figure 2.4 sets out some of the people and organisations that may be impacted by your triage.

Let's think about some of these people and how they may be affected by your triage.

- The patient
  - o May receive the most appropriate delivery of healthcare
  - o May receive advice on what to do in future
  - o May survive a life-threatening emergency because of your actions.
- The caller
  - o May receive advice (possibly life-saving) on how to manage the patient's condition
  - o May receive reassurance
  - o May be educated to help inform on any future course of action.

- Telephone-based clinicians
  - o May act on your triage to provide further care and advice.
- Other clinicians or healthcare providers
  - o May decide whether they need to provide further care or advice to a patient, based on the information you collected
  - o May tailor their care or advice based on the outcome of your triage.
- Ambulance dispatchers
  - o May prioritise ambulance resources and identify the type and speed of response required, based on your triage outcome.
- Ambulance crews
  - o May act on the information you elicit during triage to be prepared when they get to the patient
  - o May take account of the information you collected in deciding how to manage the patient.
- Commissioners
  - o May be able to better understand the level of demand for a wide range of healthcare services based on patient requirements.

- Legal representatives
  - May need to consider your actions and documentation if legal proceedings are ever needed in relation to a case you have dealt with. All information you obtain and process is considered to be legal documentation and may be used formally in any legal action or investigation that may be undertaken.

The Complexity of Telephone Triage

Carrying out telephone triage competently is a demanding skill involving a very complex process. It is dynamic – what the caller says affects how you respond, which in turn affects how the caller responds, and so on. Moreover, patients present with a myriad of different clinical situations, which can also be given a different 'flavour' by other contextual factors such as the patient's age, home circumstances, anxiety levels or any safeguarding risks. Therefore, it is impossible to come up with a list of what the 'absolutes' of any given call are.

What is essential in one call might be highly undesirable in another, for instance in some cases speaking to the patient is essential, whereas in others it would be disastrous and unsafe, such as an elderly, confused patient.

Although you will be using a system to help you assess and advise the patient, this system supports, rather than replaces, the skilled call handler. Telephone triage is demanding work and requires a lot of skill. You need to have a basic understanding of common clinical issues and terms to be able to carry out an effective assessment using the system. It is also important to understand how the system works in order to 'drive' it effectively. Good communication skills are needed to convey the questions to a wide range of callers in a wide range of situations. You must also be skilled in interpreting what callers say and in probing for further information if needed. Good listening skills are essential to ensure all relevant information is picked up. You also need to be able to provide advice with clarity and be able to judge whether it has been understood.

The lack of visual cues increases the challenge of telephone triage. Anyone involved in this area of care needs finely tuned communication skills, particularly in relation to questioning and listening, to compensate for the lack of visual cues. The ability to develop rapport is often more difficult without being able to see someone; being able to do this quickly and effectively is the mark of a skilled call handler.

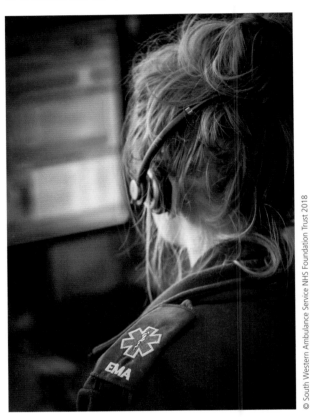

Figure 2.5 A call handler in a 999 control room

© South Western Ambulance Service NHS Foundation Trust 2018

The Importance of Clinical Decision Support Systems

A clinical decision support system (CDSS) is a tool that analyses information to help healthcare providers make effective clinical decisions. Within the context of telephone triage you may also hear CDSS referred to as 'the triage system'.

Appropriate clinical decisions involve a process where the right information is collected and analysed before reaching a decision. Within the context of telephone triage, CDSS supports effective decisions by presenting a structured set of relevant questions. This enables the right information to be collected, at the right time, in the right amount. Once enough information has been collected to decide the level and priority of care needed by the person, an outcome will be presented on the screen along with any relevant advice for the patient about what they can do to ease, minimise or manage the problem.

Time out activity – the benefits of CDSS

There are a number of benefits to using CDSS, many of which we sometimes take for granted. In highlighting these advantages, it's a useful exercise to think about how different telephone triage would be both for the patient and you, the call handler, if a decision support system wasn't in place.

Spend some time reflecting on this now before reading on.

The information will also include any relevant care advice that can be carried out to treat the problem, or prevent it deteriorating, before further care is sought.

A CDSS ensures that the assessment outcome and advice provided are all underpinned by the most reliable and current clinical evidence or research.

This ensures that the care the patient receives is safe, effective and has been well-tested. A CDSS will provide the means to assess any potential symptom that a patient could present with, in a safe and structured way that is consistent with best practice. Clearly, it would not be possible for any human being both to be able to hold all the knowledge needed to do this in their head and to use it to assess every single possible symptom in a structured and consistent way.

Decision support systems ensure that regardless of who is carrying out the assessment, the correct outcome will be reached, if used competently. This is important, because we all come to telephone triage with different knowledge, skills and backgrounds. Using an effective CDSS also means that the assessment can easily cater for different patient groups (e.g. different ages and genders) and that relevant medical conditions can be taken into account in determining the safest outcome for the patient.

A CDSS helps you, as a call handler, to control a call effectively, since the structure and flow of the questions presented gives a very specific focus at any one time. Additionally, modern-day CDSS will document the call 'automatically', vastly reducing the need to add additional documentation. This leads to a consistent, concise and adequate clinical record that can easily be shared with other healthcare providers where appropriate. On a similar point, some decision support systems 'talk' seamlessly to other systems, meaning that as well as providing a means to assess and direct patients, call handlers can make appointments or dispatch ambulances.

However, a clinical decision support system is a tool for clinical practice; like any tool, it can either be used skillfully or not. In fact, using a CDSS is a bit like driving a car. A car can be really great at getting you from A to B, but is useless without a driver. In the hands of a skilled driver, who knows the route, understands the rules and risks and has a good technique, the journey is likely to be safe (no accidents) and effective (gets you to the right place, at the right time). In the hands of a poor driver, the opposite can be true. The same could be said of decision support systems.

The Limits of Telephone Triage

Whilst telephone triage has become an important pillar in UK healthcare, it does have its limitations. The aim within telephone triage is not to diagnose the patient's problem, but to signpost them appropriately to the right form of care. Sometimes this might involve further assessment by someone with more clinical training and experience. This might be another telephone-based clinician or a professional providing further assessment in a face-to-face setting.

There is a limit to what can be achieved over the telephone because a visual assessment or physical examination is not possible. Being able to see a patient, examine them and carry out diagnostic investigations when necessary, means that it is often possible to exclude things that cannot be ruled out over the telephone. For example, it is sometimes necessary to carry out certain face-to-face examinations or investigations before being able to determine how severe an injury is.

However, this does not mean that telephone triage does not have an important part to play, simply that there is sometimes a limit to what can be done without having the patient in front of you.

Your Role as a Call Handler within Telephone Triage

Telephone triage within the context of the call handler role does not involve making diagnoses. Rather, the goal is to direct the caller to the appropriate level of care or service in a safe and timely manner while also providing self-care, life saving instructions on occasions, and risk management advice where appropriate.

The issue of diagnosis is an important one. The aim of your role is never to make a diagnosis, but rather to conduct a structured, evidence-based assessment in order to rule out potential life-threatening situations/causes for the patient's problem. This involves collecting relevant information, which is fed into the system to determine the nature and urgency of the patient's problem. Sometimes a patient will have already done an element of self-triage and may have a good idea of what care they need. Alternatively, they may have consulted with friends, relatives or work colleagues before contacting your service.

In your role as a call handler, you are asking questions or sending information to callers, which hopefully they are receiving. When the caller replies, they are sending information back to you.

This communication involves both verbal and non-verbal signals via a telephony system. However, as we have already mentioned, during telephone triage the majority of the message is verbal. It is very important to listen carefully to the words and phrases being used because you don't have the benefit of seeing what's going on with the caller.

Telephone communication removes all visual clues; therefore it is vital that you choose your words and phrases very carefully.

This whole process may sound simple; in fact, it is very complex. In addition to navigating this complex communication process, you also need to navigate the decision support system used by your organisation. The more familiar and experienced you become with the system, the more you can concentrate on the communication process.

Being able to build a picture of what the caller is describing in your mind's eye is a very valuable technique to help you retain what the patient or caller is telling you. It is easier to remember something that you've heard AND 'seen' rather than something you've only heard. So, listen to the words and images used by the caller and try to picture what they are describing.

Call Complexity and Role Boundaries

Call handlers play a pivotal role in telephone triage in England within both NHS 111 and the ambulance service, but they should not be expected to manage complex calls – this is a clinician's role. A clinician brings with them a greater level of clinical knowledge, experience and intuition, and can be held to account for their decisions by way of their professional code of conduct and registration. Of course, in order to be able to transfer the call to a clinician you need to recognise it as something which is outside of your skillset. Follow what you have been taught in training as well as any guidelines provided. It is also important to listen to your inner voice; whenever you feel out of your depth, you must seek clinical support. The point at which you feel out of your depth may be different to the point at which another call handler would start to struggle. What matters is listening to *your own* inner voice, and never struggling on to manage something which is outside of your remit, or beyond your skills and knowledge.

Call Patterns

Within telephone triage you will handle calls from people from every walk of life – different ages, genders, ethnicity, language spoken, sexual orientation, personalities, levels of ability/disability, education, social background and so on. You need to be able to deal with everyone with respect and sensitivity irrespective of their background. You also need to be able to adapt your approach according to the different needs of callers. For example, a frail, elderly hard of hearing caller requires a different approach to a mum calling about a child. A person calling about a sensitive sexual health-related issue might need a different approach to someone calling with severe breathlessness. We will talk more about this in the communication section in Chapter Three.

Irrespective of the type of service you work for, you need to be prepared to take calls of all levels of urgency. The NHS can be difficult to navigate. It is not uncommon for people to ring 999 for minor problems and NHS 111 for very urgent medical issues. For example, data from NHS Digital (2017) show that:

- Calls to 999 and 111 are received about all age groups from birth to very old age. However, calls about adult females are the most common. About a quarter of all calls concern people under 16 years of age.

- The busiest times of the week often tend to be Saturday and Sunday with twice as many calls as during a week day. This obviously has implications for you, as it is likely that weekend working will form a significant part of your role.

- The busiest hours of the day are between 5pm and 8pm on weekdays and between 8am and 11am during the weekend. This is also relevant to your role, because it means that you will likely be required to work evenings a lot of the time.

- Telephone triage is also unpredictable. Anybody can call about anything. This has implications for you as a call handler because it means you must remain alert and focused at all times, whilst being quite agile in how you respond to different things. Part of what allows you to do this is becoming skilled at leaving each call behind before you take another one. This important habit will be discussed in more detail later within the book.

- The following scenarios show how varied calls to telephone triage services can be, ranging from simple and minor conditions through to complex or life-threatening emergencies. Do remember, though, that you will be using an assessment tool which will guide you through the process. You are not expected to memorise the process.

Scenarios

Scenario 1 – Bob

Bob is a 53-year-old man. He has just returned from a run and starts to complain of 'indigestion'. His wife urges him to call 111 so they can find the closest pharmacy to get some indigestion medication.

Although Bob plays down his symptoms, the call handler establishes that he has pain in the centre and left of his chest. He carries out an assessment and it becomes apparent that the pain feels like a heavy weight or tight band. Bob says it feels a bit like 'an elephant sitting on me'.

The outcome is an emergency ambulance which Bob initially refuses because he thinks it is unnecessary. However, the call handler relates back to Bob the symptoms he has described and persuades him that it would be a good idea for the ambulance crew to come and assess him. He agrees and when the crew arrive they carry out various investigations. It is suspected that Bob may have had a heart attack and he is taken to hospital. Here it is confirmed that he has, in fact, had a heart attack and he receives appropriate care to help him recover from this serious event.

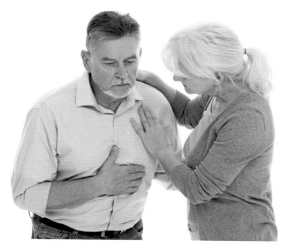

Figure 2.6 Bob calls 111 to complain of 'indigestion'

© PIKSEL/ iStock

Scenario 2 – Sarah

Sarah is a 52 year-old woman. She called 999 following a fall at home and is now finding it almost impossible to walk. She feels she would be unable to drive herself to the emergency department, so thought it best to call an ambulance.

The call handler excluded any life-threatening symptoms and established that Sarah's pain seemed to be getting worse. However, there were no other worrying features. The outcome of the triage was a recommendation from the call handler that Sarah attended the nearby minor injury unit (MIU) within the next four hours. It is explained that they will be able to provide the care Sarah needs, rather than her needing to go to the emergency department. Sarah explained that she could not drive herself to the MIU and that was why she had phoned an ambulance. The call handler explained that as long as Sarah managed to get to the MIU in the next four hours that would be fine and asked whether Sarah could perhaps ask a friend, relative or neighbour to take her. Reluctantly, Sarah agreed to phone her sister to ask for a lift.

Sarah's sister took her to the MIU shortly afterwards and Sarah was seen within 30 minutes of arriving. It was established that she had suffered a sprain which would get better with the help of rest, ice, compression and elevation at home.

Scenario 3 – Lauren

Lauren is a three-year-old child. She has been complaining of earache so her dad decides to call 111. The call handler rules out any serious issues and establishes that the earache has been present for three hours and that Lauren doesn't have a fever. The outcome of the triage is to refer the call to a 111 clinician for some advice about how to manage the problem at home. Lauren's dad says he would prefer that she saw the doctor and had some antibiotics.

The call is transferred to a 111 clinician who asks a few further questions for clarification. The clinician agrees that the problem can be managed at home. She talks Lauren's dad through some basic advice about how to ease the pain and reassures him that earache often gets better without any treatment. Lauren's dad repeats that he would like her to have antibiotics, at which point, the clinician takes some time to explain why that's not necessary and could, in fact, be counterproductive. She reassures Lauren's dad that he can call back anytime if things do not seem to be improving.

Lauren's dad gives her some painkillers and continues to do this regularly, according to the instructions on the packet. Lauren seems to brighten enormously and within a day her earache has resolved.

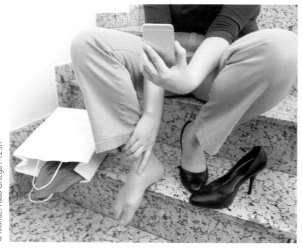

© Manuel Faba Ortega / 123rf

Figure 2.7 Unable to drive herself to the emergency department Sarah is advised to ask her sister for a lift

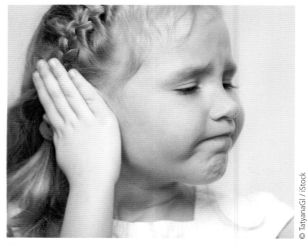

© TatyanaGl / iStock

Figure 2.8 Lauren has been complaining of earache and the call is referred to a 111 clinician for some advice on managing the problem at home

Scenario 4 – Aaron

Aaron is a four-month-old baby who has been crying on and off for the last two hours. His mum Samantha is 19 years old and this is her first baby. She is extremely anxious and is worried that Aaron's distress is being caused by something serious. She has been trying to get hold of her health visitor for the last 20 minutes, but keeps getting an answerphone message. It is 6pm, so it is likely that the health visiting team is unavailable at this time. Samantha decides she cannot take any more and phones 999.

The call handler can hear Aaron crying in the background and can sense Samantha's anxiety. She uses a reassuring voice to try and get Samantha to calm down a little. The assessment rules out anything life-threatening; at the end of the assessment, Samantha is advised that Aaron needs to be seen within primary care in the next two hours. The call handler is able to make an appointment with the GP Out of Hours service and Samantha walks Aaron there in his pram. By the time they arrive, Aaron is asleep; however, the GP examines him and advises that he is probably a little constipated. He gives some advice about how to manage this. He notices that Aaron looks a little underweight and, after agreeing it with Samantha, he leaves a message for the health visiting team asking for someone to visit them at home.

Scenario 5 – Liviu

Liviu is a 67-year-old man. He has been having rectal bleeding for the past three weeks but has kept it to himself. He is worried his wife might want him to go to hospital. However, the problem has got worse and his wife has guessed what is going on. She has insisted that he contact 111.

The call handler tries to carry out an assessment of the problem. However, Liviu suffers from hearing loss so the assessment takes a considerable time and the call handler has to speak slowly and clearly. The assessment determines that Liviu needs to go straight to his nearest emergency department. As a result, Liviu is seen a week later by a specialist and a diagnosis of bowel cancer is made. He receives surgery and a course of chemotherapy.

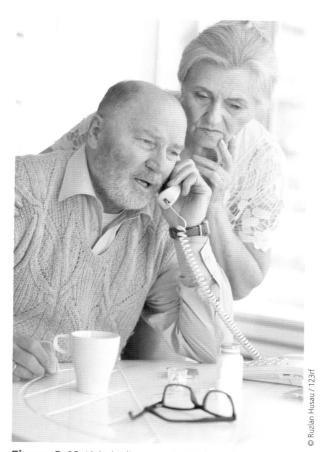

© Ruzlan Husau / 123rf

Figure 2.10 Liviu is diagnosed with bowel cancer after seeing a specialist

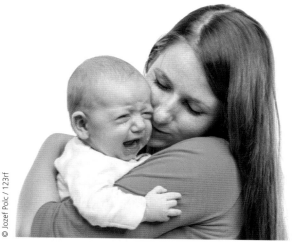

© Jozef Polc / 123rf

Figure 2.9 Aaron's mother is extremely anxious that his crying is caused by something serious

Scenario 6 – James

James is a university student who is invited to a party by friends. Whilst at the party he takes some Class A drugs. He is found collapsed by his friend Nirpal who calls 999.

The call handler establishes that James isn't breathing. Nirpal is instructed how to carry out resuscitation until the crew arrive. The crew arrive within about four minutes and are able to take over from Nirpal who is becoming exhausted.

James receives a series of electric shocks to try and restart his heart. The crew report that James regains a pulse and after some time, he is transported to hospital. James is discharged several days later and makes a full recovery.

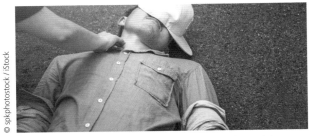

Figure 2.11 James collapses at a party after taking Class A drugs

Scenario 7 – Hugo

Hugo is a 30-year-old man who has recently been through a traumatic marriage separation. He has also just found out that he is going to be made redundant. He has suffered with episodes of depression in the past and has recently been suffering with very low mood and difficulty sleeping.

Today, his lodger returned home to find that Hugo had attempted suicide by cutting his wrist. He is conscious but bleeding quite heavily. The lodger phones 999 and Hugo speaks to the call handler. He becomes angry and aggressive, but the call handler remains calm and warm in her approach. She has difficulty understanding what

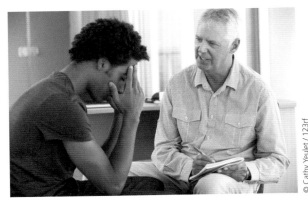

Figure 2.12 Hugo is assessed by a mental health crisis team

Hugo is saying as he does not seem to be making sense.

An ambulance is dispatched and, after his wounds have been dealt with, Hugo is taken to the emergency department. The crew explain to Hugo that he needs to be seen urgently for the sake of his physical and mental health, although they explain that they cannot force him. Hugo agrees but says that he will not stay there long. In the emergency department he is assessed by a mental health crisis team. He is discharged home into the care of a relative and receives ongoing support from mental health services.

Scenario 8 – Rumbi

Rumbi is a 30-year-old woman who originates from East Africa. She has been experiencing abdominal pain for two days and has been told by a friend to call 111 for help.

Rumbi has a vague understanding of the English language and the call handler finds it difficult to understand what she's saying. She establishes the language that Rumbi speaks and gets her permission to get an interpreter on the line. The assessment is conducted through the interpreter and Rumbi is advised to be seen at the walk-in centre close to Rumbi's flat.

Rumbi is examined and found to have constipation. She is given advice about how to manage this, and prevent it re-occurring.

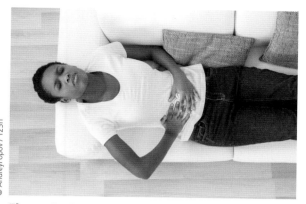

© AndreyPopov / 123rf

Figure 2.13 Rumbi has been experiencing stomach pain for two days

Summary

The contribution telephone triage makes to a patient's care cannot be underestimated and your role as a call handler within this is crucial. Although you are not a clinician it is likely that your input will directly affect any clinical care that the patient does ultimately receive.

Reference

Data supplied from NHS Digital, 2017, via the Intelligent Data Tool.

Chapter 3: Telephone Communication

Learning Objectives

By the end of this chapter you will be able to:

- Explain the importance of good communication within healthcare including telephone triage
- Describe a model of communication
- Explain the essentials of how to control the flow and pace of a call
- Describe skilled questioning
- Explain active listening over the telephone
- Explain methods and techniques for building rapport
- State how to balance warmth and professionalism
- Explain how to demonstrate respect and sensitivity
- Describe how to negotiate with callers
- Summarise the essentials of conflict resolution within telephone triage.

Introduction

Effective communication is the foundation of skilled telephone triage and is at the core of the call handling role. Skilled communication over the telephone, especially in a frequently high-stress and highly emotive environment, is something that requires development and practice. Inter-personal communication forms a fundamental aspect of our daily lives. As such, we rarely stop to think about how we do it. This lack of focused attention on how we communicate is perhaps reflected by the fact that more complaints are received about poor communication within the NHS than any other factor [HSCIC, 2016].

At its simplest level, communication is simply the act of transferring information from a sender to a receiver. However, the process is actually very complex. We communicate using different channels such as verbal, non-verbal and written. Communication involves the 'sender' encoding or translating a message into a form that is appropriate to the communication channel. For face-to-face communication, this is usually language and non-verbal gestures or responses. Once the message has been 'sent', the receiver needs to 'decode' or interpret it. In order for communication to be successful, the receiver needs to understand the message sent, but as with any complex process, particularly one where much of what happens is automatic and unconscious, there is great potential for things to go wrong. Figure 3.1 below presented by Corcoran (2013) shows how communication is a cyclical process where understanding and feedback to the sender form an important part of the process. Checking that the message given has been understood through feedback from the receiver is fundamental to ensure that messages have been understood in the way in which they were intended [Corcoran, 2013].

Within telephone triage, there is perhaps even more potential for things to go wrong, because the absence of visual stimuli means that both the sender and receiver need to employ different techniques to ensure the right information is sent and received.

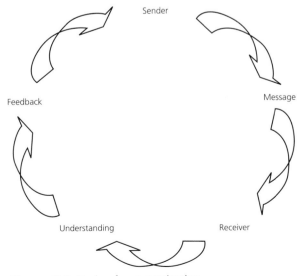

Figure 3.1 Cycle of communication

There is evidence to show that non-verbal communication often conveys a much more powerful message than the words we use. If the verbal message and the non-verbal message do not match, we tend to believe the non-verbal message. Over the telephone however, much of the non-verbal language that we normally use becomes redundant. We cannot use a great deal of non-verbal communication over the telephone, so it is very different to communicating in person. We cannot rely on being able to see each other and all the information that this provides, which means we need to be a very skilled verbal communicator. Tone of voice and the stress you put on different words are also very important. The same words delivered in different tones and with different emphasis can have an entirely different meaning. Try reading out this sentence in different tones and with the emphasis on just one of each of the different words, and see what the impact is: 'I am really enjoying reading this book'. So, for example, putting stress on the 'I' part of the sentence gives it a different flavour to when we place emphasis on the 'this' part of the sentence.

Within telephone triage, there are other factors to consider which can interfere with the transmission and understanding of the message. One of these factors is noise. In practical terms, this could be a patient calling from a mobile phone with poor reception or a loud television. It may also mean distractions such as a screaming child or someone arguing in the background. A busy call centre will also produce 'noise' such as lots of people talking on the phone to callers or even colleagues talking to each other, which can also be a considerable distraction.

Within telephone triage you need to be especially skilled in quickly reading a situation and, if necessary, adapting the way you communicate. You need to be able to recognise when the situation demands a different type of communication and change the approach accordingly.

Controlling the Pace and Flow of the Call

Keeping control of a call can be difficult but it is an important part of ensuring a safe outcome for a patient. Controlling a call requires the ability to steer the consultation to the best outcome for the patient in the most direct way possible. It does not mean being domineering, rude, dispassionate or leading. Reaching the best outcome in the most direct way has obvious benefits for the patient, the call handler and the organisation. Patients' experience of well-controlled calls tends to be more positive; they sense that they are having their problem dealt with safely, professionally and effectively. This matters, because when a patient's impression of the service is good they are more likely to use it again and recommend it to others.

When a call is controlled poorly and the patient is allowed to give too much information, the call handler can easily lose sight of the most important clinical information with the obvious risk of not reaching the most appropriate outcome. Longer calls also mean that other potential users of the service may spend longer waiting to get through, which may jeopardise their health.

Speaking to the Patient

Triage is often more effective when it is carried out directly with the patient; introducing a third party can often create a 'Chinese whispers' effect. Talking with the patient also enables you to evaluate for yourself important factors such as the nature of the person's breathing, speech patterns, comprehension and so on. With first-party calls, certain questions don't need to be asked such as whether the person is very breathless because you can 'hear' the answer to the question. Thus, first-party triage is often quicker and more accurate.

Patients may also reveal important information to a call handler that they are reluctant or unwilling to discuss with friends or family.

It is vital to remember that there are situations where speaking to the patient is appropriate and others where it is not. It would usually not be appropriate to ask to speak to someone who is in an obviously life-threatening situation. Nor would it be appropriate to conduct an assessment with someone who is confused or a very young child. You must exercise judgement as to how strenuously to pursue talking to the patient rather than the caller. Every call is different and requires skilled judgement on the part of the person handling it (Figure 3.2).

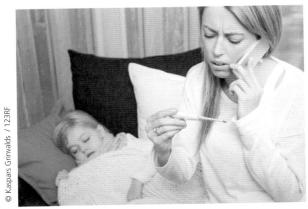

© Kaspars Grinvalds / 123RF

Figure 3.2 Sometimes it will be necessary to speak to a third party rather than directly with the patient

The Impact of Emotion on Call Control

Controlling a call where the caller is particularly emotional can present additional challenges, but it is often these calls that most require effective call control. For example, a parent ringing about a child who has stopped breathing is bound to be extremely distressed. In this situation, your ability to deal with this distress and control the call effectively could quite literally mean the difference between life and death.

When someone appears to be experiencing very strong emotions such as anger, frustration or anxiety, it can help to look beyond what they are saying and how they are saying it and focus instead on what has brought them to call. Underneath any strong emotion is usually some kind of 'need'. Often with negative emotions, there is an unmet need. It is our job to try and uncover this need, acknowledge it and respond appropriately. This can help you adapt the way you respond allowing you to take back control of the situation, which ultimately benefits the patient.

If a caller suddenly becomes highly emotional during the course of a call, think about what you have said and how you have said it, to determine reasons for their change in behaviour. It is quite possibly a lack of mutual understanding that has led to their frustration which, in turn, has led to them changing their tactics. Call control is about steering the pace and content of the call effectively, not about 'wrestling' it from the caller.

Setting the Scene

An important part of controlling the call involves clearly but concisely setting out the process which you will be taking the caller through. Callers are more likely to engage in and cooperate with the process if they understand it. This is particularly the case with less urgent calls where a longer string of questions is required. However, there are clearly some situations when there is no time to explain the call process (e.g. when someone has stopped breathing). Again, judgement about the situation is required.

Directing the Flow and Pace of the Call

An essential part of telephone triage is guiding the caller to provide the right kind of information, in the right quantity, at the right time. It may mean slowing the caller down, moving them on to a different point or stopping a particular stream of information which is not required.

The speed of the call must be consistent with the requirements of the situation. For example, it is important to rule out any threat to life rapidly; if a call is potentially life-threatening or urgent, this rapid pace needs to be maintained throughout. However, this does not mean speeding up so much that the quality of the outcome is compromised. Responding to a caller's needs might include slowing down a little for a particularly distressed caller, so as to respond appropriately to their emotional state.

Controlling the flow and pace of a call involves the combined skills of being able to talk, listen, assimilate information and use all relevant IT and telephony equipment without sounding mechanistic, stilted or computer driven. This takes time to develop, but is possible with experience.

The issue of whether to refer to the clinical decision support system (CDSS) you are using is an interesting one. Whilst callers generally understand that a computer is being used, people don't like to feel 'processed', especially when it comes to important issues concerning their health. It is best to avoid phrases which overemphasise the contribution of a computer such as 'the system's telling me … ', 'it's coming up with advice to … ' or 'it says here you should … '. This does not mean that you should ever be dishonest if asked whether you are using a computer, just that you should not undermine what is in fact a very skilled 'human' process. If this situation does arise, it would be worth stressing how the system you are using helps you to provide up-to-date and high-quality care and advice.

Five tips for effective call control

1. Using the caller's name

Sometimes this can be all it takes to gain control of a call. Using the caller's name can be enough to stop a person in their tracks and listen to what you have to say.

2. Recognising if the caller doesn't understand something

Callers may be confused or frustrated by some of the questions they are asked. Explaining the process at the outset is helpful, but you may also need to stop and explain the purpose of specific questions if you can sense that the caller has not understood something.

3. Repetitive persistence

The idea here is to repeat a phrase with exactly the same calm, caring but firm intonation with the intention of getting the caller to mirror your demeanour. An example might be 'Sir, I need to make sure that she's breathing so that I can get her the right care and then you can tell me more about her pain'. This can be very effective when dealing with highly emotional callers and is commonly used in 999 settings.

The key to this technique is staying very calm. Usually, repeating yourself three times should be enough. If you have repeated yourself three times and not gained control of the call, a different approach may need to be taken. This is not an effective technique if the problem is that the caller does not understand a specific question. If this was the case you would need to rephrase it, rather than just keep restating it. This technique is about gaining cooperation in a calm way or about cutting through strong emotion that has stalled the process.

4. Polite interruption

It is possible to interrupt in a way that is polite and friendly – sometimes this is necessary if you are not getting the information you need. This does need to be done carefully so as not to appear rude or give the impression you are not listening. A good method is to interrupt the caller's flow of information by continuing their sentence in the same pitch and pace. It also helps to pick up on the words that they've used to demonstrate that you have listened.

Once you have control of the conversation you can then lead it in the direction that you need to go. An example might be:

CALLER: 'Yes, I take lots of other tablets that it might be useful for you to know about, such as …'
CALL HANDLER: 'Ah okay, so you take quite a lot of medication. Let me ask you a few more questions and then if I need to know about your medication you can tell me.'

5. Keeping the caller informed throughout the call

As well as informing callers about the process of triage at the start of a call, it's useful to keep them informed of the different stages as you go through them. Without this, it can sometimes seem like a never-ending string of questions with no obvious purpose. Saying something like: 'That's the end of my questions. I do have some advice about things that might help, and then I can tell you what options you have for your next steps.' This only takes a moment and, if it stops someone becoming frustrated or disengaged, it can actually save time. The same applies if you need to put them on hold for any reason; this can feel bewildering for a caller if they do not understand what is happening.

Another example might be if you were staying on the line to provide support during a cardiac arrest. It can feel like the ambulance is taking a long time to arrive, but reminding the caller that help is coming as quickly as possibly can help to reassure them.

Skilled Questioning

Telephone triage using decision support systems is essentially a series of questions to be answered. It stands to reason that being able to ask these questions effectively is a vital skill. Effective questioning is quite a complex task and within a telephone triage environment it can be broken down into two broad areas:

1. Conveying a question skilfully.
2. Probing for more information if the initial question did not elicit the information required or more detail is needed.

Conveying Questions Skilfully

It is essential that each question is phrased in a way that communicates accurately the intended clinical meaning. The way the question is asked should mean that none of the clinical meaning is lost or altered, even if this meaning is quite subtle. Whilst retaining the clinical meaning, it is essential to phrase questions in a way that callers can understand. It would be entirely possible to convey the meaning of a question accurately, but have a situation where the caller does not understand what is being asked, which clearly renders the question useless. Therefore, skill is needed in phrasing questions so that they are easily understood. This means that you need to be adaptable according to the needs of the situation and to read the situation well. In rephrasing a question you may need to use supplementary information derived from the system you're using or from your training, to guide you in forming alternative ways of asking the same question.

Jargon is terminology that relates to a specific activity, profession or group. In the context of telephone triage it means avoiding the use of medical jargon or terminology which is service or system specific. An example of medical jargon would be 'haematemesis' rather than vomiting blood. Of course, some patients are knowledgeable about their condition and may themselves use medical terms. In these circumstances it would be acceptable to adopt the term used by the patient or caller, but it would be essential to check out the meaning attached to this term by the person using it, before adopting it yourself. For example, if a patient referred to their 'epigastric area', even if you knew exactly where this was, you would need to ensure that the caller was using this term correctly.

In forming questions, it is important not to use questions which have the potential to 'lead' callers into providing certain responses. The questions listed in Table 3.1 are examples of leading questions, along with more appropriate ways of asking each question.

Table 3.1 Leading and straightforward questions

Leading questions	Straightforward questions
It didn't start suddenly, did it?	Did it start suddenly?
He's not brought up blood?	Has he brought up any blood?
No problems with her breathing?	Any problems with her breathing?

Not all callers will be led by such questions, but some will. Callers more likely to be led include those that are distracted, anxious or have communication difficulties. However, as with any aspect of triage, this also requires judgement. In some situations, questions like those listed above do have a place. For example, if a caller had already said at the start of the call that their headache started gradually, it would be entirely acceptable to clarify this by asking *'It didn't start suddenly, did it?'* This would signal to the caller that they had been listened to earlier. Another situation where this type of question can be appropriate is where it seems extremely unlikely that the situation being asked about would apply. For example, if someone rang to say they had hit their thumb with a hammer it would be extremely unlikely that they were suffering from major blood loss and also extremely unlikely that they wouldn't have mentioned this already. It would therefore be acceptable to rule this out by asking *'There's no heavy blood loss is there?'*

Obtaining Adequate Information to Answer Each Question

Probing for further information is one of the most critical skills needed in telephone triage. One definition of the verb 'to probe' is to 'ask questions or try to discover facts' [Collins Online Dictionary, 2017]. Probing within the context of the role of a call handler involves using very specific and focused techniques to ascertain additional information about the caller's situation. Usually, probing takes the form of asking very focused questions, but posing an open question asking a caller to explain something in more detail is also a form of probing.

Callers do not know what information is needed by the system to deliver an appropriate outcome. The responsibility for gathering the appropriate information always remains with the call handler. Additionally, human nature means that callers can, at times, be vague, unclear and inconsistent. This can often be the case when someone is hurt or unwell, in pain or anxious.

Probing questions are, in essence, follow-up questions that ask for additional information. They may encourage the caller either to expand upon or be more specific about what they have said. It is not possible to be skilled within telephone triage without being skilled at probing as the majority of calls will, at some point, require this. Callers cannot be expected to know what information is needed. It is the responsibility of the call handler to ask questions that are phrased in such a way that callers are able to provide that information.

Probing is a vital skill throughout the whole call. It is often needed at the outset to establish the reason for the call or the presence of any life-threatening problems. It is needed during the symptom assessment and it may be needed once an outcome has been reached, if there seems to be resistance to this advice. Sometimes, during the assessment process, a caller may casually mention a previously undisclosed symptom that could potentially change the whole assessment. For example they might mention that the chest pain they are experiencing only came on after a fall, or they may equally have been reporting a fall, but had not mentioned that it had been preceded by chest pain. New information such as this would require a little probing, and potentially a change to the route taken through the decision support system you are using. To be skilled at probing, you need to recognise when it is necessary to obtain further information and must then form effective questions to ensure you get the necessary information.

It is also essential to realise when probing is not needed. This includes situations where ample information has been provided or where it is clear that even an endless amount of probing would not get a clear answer to a question. When you are repeatedly struggling to get the information you need, it may be necessary to seek clinical advice or to pass the call on to a clinician.

Knowing when to probe

You should consider probing further:
- If you get a confusing answer from the caller. Is this because of a confusing question? Can you resolve this by rephrasing the question?
- To make sure you understand what the caller is saying. Never make assumptions. Probe if you are not satisfied you've got the correct answers to your questions.
- To ensure that all elements of a question are answered. This might mean asking all parts of a question. For example, if there is a timescale

included in the question, you must know if the symptoms have occurred during that period in order to answer the question accurately.
- If you don't understand the caller's response.
- Only when necessary – if you're comfortable that the caller completely understood, and you have a full and adequate response that you can understand, then there's probably no need to probe. Probing for no reason does not add value to the call and can complicate and lengthen the call unnecessarily.

How to probe skilfully:
- You need to understand exactly what the question is asking.
- Listen, both to the verbal cues and the non-verbal cues such as hesitation and pauses. These can be indicators of a lack of caller understanding, which is your responsibility to address through further questioning.
- Be careful not to change the clinical meaning of the questions if you rephrase something. This will help to ensure that the caller understands what you are asking of them, whilst the essence of the question remains the same.
- Reflect on the response the caller has given as a way of probing. An example of this would be 'Do you mean the pain is bad when it comes, but that it isn't there all the time?'
- Avoid using leading questions as a form of probing. Callers may want to give you answers they 'think' you want. So, for example, by phrasing a question 'You haven't had … have you?', the caller may inadvertently answer incorrectly in an effort to 'please' you by giving you the answer they think you want.
- Be resourceful. Do not just accept the information if you think the caller has not understood or answered the question. For example, when asking if someone is warm to touch, get someone to actually feel the person's chest or abdomen if you are in any doubt about the answer you have been given.

Active Listening

Listening is the ability to accurately receive and interpret messages. It is a crucial part of communication. Without the ability to listen effectively, messages are easily misunderstood;

communication breaks down and the sender of the message can easily become frustrated or irritated. Hearing refers to the sounds that you hear, whereas listening requires more than that: it requires focus. Listening means paying attention not only to the story, but also how it is told. This includes the use of language and voice but also non-verbal cues. Even though non-verbal communication is limited over the telephone, it does still play a part. For example, if a caller repeatedly hesitates and pauses, it may indicate that they do not really understand what is being asked.

Given all the listening we do, you would think we would be really good at it. In fact, we're not. Most humans, unless hearing impaired, can hear fairly well but many of us do not really know how to listen. Studies show that we retain a dismal 25–50% of what we hear. That means that when you talk to your boss, colleagues, patients or spouse for 10 minutes, they only retain 2½–5 minutes of the conversation!

Listening is not a skill usually taught in school, even though it is fundamental to learning, but it is a skill that can be broken down and taught. Some people are naturally good at listening, but most of us need to learn and practice.

Active listening is a structured way of listening and responding with the aim of fully understanding the intended message. It is not just about passively receiving information – the response to the message is also important. So active listening is about much more than just the passive receiving of information – the response to the message is very important.

Active listening is hard work, but it is absolutely essential to your role. When using a CDSS, you effectively act as the system's ears. The system can't 'hear' what the caller says, but the caller's responses must be fed into the system so it can do its job. Therefore, excellent listening skills are vital to be able to pick up the information needed to drive the direction of the assessment.

Listening and Retaining Information

Within telephone triage it is important to listen to *what* is being said as well as *how* it is being said. It is also vital to pick up on everything else that is communicated by the caller, aside from the actual words they use. This includes the caller's

demeanour, for instance do they sound breathless, confused, disorientated, in pain or weak? It also means picking up on things like speech patterns and pauses or vague responses, as well as being alert for signs of fear, frustration, anger and anxiety.

Part of the skill of listening, involves picking up on relevant background noise. For example:

- Is there a child crying in the background?
- Is the patient moaning in pain in the background?
- Are there sounds of violence or disturbance in the background?

With all these cues, it is important to 'check out' what you have heard rather than making an assumption about what it might mean. An example of this would be asking 'Is that (patient's name) I can hear moaning in the background?' If it were indeed the patient moaning, it might give you some idea about their degree of pain.

Active listening is about so much more than just 'hearing' the information. It involves remembering and using the information you have heard. This information can be anything from the person's name, to their personal circumstances, to the clinical details given. It is vital to actively listen from beginning to end, as important information may be provided at any point. Indeed, it is often towards the end of a call, that significant information emerges; it is vital not to be 'closed' to this information just because it did not emerge earlier.

Demonstrating that you are Listening

In a normal face-to-face conversation, we use eye contact, nods and smiles to show the other person that we are listening, but obviously these are redundant over the phone. The person cannot see you nodding so you need to use 'verbal nods' such as 'uh-uh', 'right' 'yes' 'okay' 'I see' etc. Use these carefully, as some people have a tendency to overuse the same verbal nod which can become irritating or sound a little robotic.

Remember – and use – the details people have already given to you. These can be anything from the person's name, to their personal circumstances, to the clinical details given. You can only pick these up though, if you're paying attention!

We can show the caller we are listening, by asking appropriate questions. Obviously the system you are using will provide questions for you to ask, but this does not remove your responsibility to conduct the assessment with a common sense approach. If someone has already given you all the information you need to fully answer a question, there is often no need to ask it. In asking a question where all the information needed has already been given, you are not demonstrating to the caller that you have listened. For example, if someone phones and says 'She's rolling around in agony at the moment with the pain' you do not need to ask if the patient has any pain.

Using appropriate responses to clarify information is important in terms of demonstrating that you are listening. If someone has already mentioned something which you need more details about, you will need to clarify. The way you do this should demonstrate that you heard it in the first place. For example, let's imagine someone phones about a patient and says 'they're having problems breathing and a sharp pain in their chest'. Once you reach a question asking about the presence of any chest pain, you need to make sure the question is 'framed' in such a way that demonstrates you picked up on the presence of a sharp pain in the patient's chest. It would not sound like you had been listening if you were to ask 'have they got any chest pain?' as the person has already told you this. It would be better to paraphrase or reflect back what had already been said, for example 'You said he had a sharp pain in his chest. Is that the only pain in his chest he has?' Techniques such as paraphrasing are a useful way to demonstrate that you are listening. Another example would be 'When you said he was "bringing up blood", does that mean he is coughing it up or that he has vomited blood?' Again, this demonstrates listening, whilst allowing for probing about the situation.

Improving Listening Skills

It's vital to give each call all of your attention. Many adverse events in the health service are as a result of the patient or their family not being properly listened to. Be deliberate with your listening and remind yourself constantly that your goal is to truly hear what the other person is saying.

Top tips for effective listening

1. Stop talking

   '*If we were supposed to talk more than we listen, we would have two tongues and one ear*' – Mark Twain.

   When a caller is talking, really listen to what they are saying. Avoid interrupting (unless it's necessary for call control), talking over them or finishing their sentences. When the caller has finished talking, you may need to clarify to ensure you have received their message accurately.

2. Remove distractions

   Before each call, remind yourself to relax and focus on the caller. The human brain is easily distracted by other thoughts so before you take each call, take a few seconds to commit to putting other concerns out of your mind. Take active steps to reduce distractions during the call. This can be tricky in a busy call centre environment. Focus your gaze away from distractions such as colleagues, the window and wall boards, etc.

3. Put the caller at ease

   Ensure that the caller is aware that they are free to speak. Use verbal nods to encourage them to continue and remember their needs and concerns.

4. Keep an open mind

   Try to understand the caller's point of view. Look at issues from their perspective and let go of preconceived ideas. Having an open mind enables us to fully take on board what the caller is saying.

5. Be patient

   Recognise that some calls may take a little longer, for instance those regarding a mental health concern or a particularly sensitive issue.

6. Avoid personal prejudice

   Try to be impartial. Do not become irritated and try not to let the person's habits or mannerisms distract you from their message. Callers will communicate in very different ways. Some are more nervous or shy than others, some have strong regional accents and, for some callers, English will not be their first language. Focus on what is being said and try to look beyond the various styles of delivery. Some callers may display strong emotions and may seem aggressive or angry. However, it is important to remember that they have called your service for help and it is your responsibility to try and provide it. Make sure you are aware of your local policy in relation to dealing with challenging calls.

7. Listen to the whole message

    Volume and tone both add to what someone is saying. Listen carefully to these to get a feel for the emphasis of what is being said. One of the most difficult aspects of listening over the telephone is the ability to link together pieces of information in order to form a coherent 'picture' of the overall situation. With good concentration and letting go of distractions, this process of 'picture building' becomes easier. Sometimes, this information is drip fed, whilst at other times it is delivered in a deluge. Both situations can be challenging; if you ever struggle to piece together the information, it is important to seek guidance from a clinician.

8. Rephrasing and probing

    If a caller does not seem to understand what is being asked of them you may need to rephrase the question to make the message clearer. Again, if you are ever in any doubt about the rephrasing of a question, always seek assistance from a clinician.

Establishing Rapport

Building rapport with a caller is important because it facilitates an easier exchange of information; the effective two-way exchange of information is what telephone triage is all about. Rapport involves creating a relationship of mutual understanding and trust. It does not necessarily mean agreeing with everything the other person says, but it does mean trying to get on the same wavelength as the caller. It takes skill to build rapport quickly, which is what is required with telephone triage. Skilled verbal communication (the actual words used) as well as skilled non-verbal communication (the way the words are used) is essential for effective rapport building.

The first consideration when trying to build rapport is to sound natural. This can be trickier when you are referring to questions on the screen or using a script but this does not have to make you sound robotic. Being familiar with the content of the system, and any scripts you are given, will help you to use them in a more natural, fluent way. Your aim should be to become an expert in how you use your voice, with the intention of always sounding warm, natural and friendly, whilst being professional and also firm when needed. Listening to your own calls can be a really useful development activity, particularly in relation to how you use your voice.

Time out activity – using your voice skilfully

Over the telephone, it is vital that the voice conveys a genuine desire to help as well as the words we use. This is called congruence. For example, the phrase 'I'm trying to help you' can convey several different messages depending on where the emphasis is placed and the tone used.

Try it out now, using different tones and placing the emphasis on different words.

Another important practice when trying to develop rapport within telephone triage is to make sure you actively acknowledge the person's need. You must make sure you understand what has prompted the call. Something has obviously caused the caller to contact the service, be this pain, sickness, a request for a visit, a need for information, etc. Unless you understand exactly what made the person call, it can be hard to build rapport.

Acknowledge that you have heard this need and be honest about what you can do. Actively refer to the patient's concerns in the language you use. Recognising a need might not mean you can solve it, but it is still important to acknowledge the patient's concerns and explain what you can do to respond. Side-stepping around things just makes people feel you're not listening, don't understand or don't care.

Time out activity – consider the following scenario

A man falls off a ladder and hurts his ankle. In the course of your assessment, you discover that the reason he fell was because he blacked out. He is not sure what caused the blackout and is not particularly concerned about it. He is, however, very concerned about his ankle because it is very painful.

It is, of course, right that the blackout becomes the main focus of your assessment because it may have a serious cause. Taking a few moments to explain why you are concerned about the blackout, as well as his ankle, demonstrates that you have acknowledged the reason he has called. This may prevent him feeling that his real problem is being ignored, which should ultimately help you develop rapport. Rapport is important because without it, callers may be reluctant to engage fully in the assessment process or to follow your advice.

Balancing Warmth and Professionalism

When we access any kind of service, we have a right to expect the person providing that service to be polite. When accessing healthcare, we also have a right to expect to be treated with care and compassion. A key skill within any area of healthcare is to maintain an appropriate balance between the need to be professional and the need to respond to the patient/caller in a warm and compassionate way. On a very basic level, the interaction that goes on is between two human beings, one of whom has some kind of problem and another who has the ability to help in some way. Often people are contacting your service with deeply intimate, worrying or serious issues; it is important that in providing healthcare, you do this with warmth and compassion. This does not mean becoming overly familiar with the caller or patient, but it does mean relating to them as a fellow human being who is 'hurting' or suffering in some way. Whatever the problem, it can help to put yourself in the caller's shoes or to imagine someone you love dearly in their position. Your voice is one of your most powerful tools in conveying a genuine sense of care and compassion.

Within the health service, we all have a responsibility to be professional. The essence of being professional means carrying out your role with regard for appropriate standards. It includes factors such as avoiding being overly familiar or informal with callers. It also includes using suitable language. In order to demonstrate a polite and professional manner it is vital to acknowledge the nature of your role: you are providing a service to the patient, not the other way around. So, whilst callers may be poor communicators, rude or difficult, this is never an excuse for you to be unprofessional or demonstrate bad manners. Of course, some callers can be very challenging, particularly if they are in pain, anxious or suffering deeply in some way. However, this is the nature of your role – you are bound to come into contact with people that are difficult to deal with. When you handle a particularly challenging call, make sure you get adequate support and debriefing if needed. Talking these situations through with someone can help you make sense of the experience or put it in perspective: this will stop you from carrying the event with you, possibly into the next call or into your personal life.

Respect and Sensitivity

Communicating sensitively involves demonstrating empathy and compassion for the situation as the caller/patient is experiencing it, as well as appropriate regard for their emotions and feelings. Empathy is the ability to imagine how another person is feeling – putting yourself in their shoes. It is different from sympathy, which is more about feeling sorry for someone without really trying to understand how they are feeling. Within healthcare, empathy is really about being able to imagine a person's situation, whilst not forgetting that you have a job to do.

The call handler should demonstrate respect for both the caller and patient. On a fundamental level, respect means showing regard and appreciation for the worth of someone or something. It also means that there is a demonstration of acceptance of the person, despite any apparent differences. These can include differences involving religion, culture, race, sexual orientation, age, gender and so on. In essence, respect is about treating someone the way you would wish to be treated. We live in an incredibly diverse population and it is important that you treat everyone, irrespective of any apparent differences between you and them, with respect and with a sensitive understanding of their situation.

Negotiating with Callers

Negotiation is a discussion intended to produce an agreement where each party initially has an opposing view/requirement. Everybody negotiates: at work, at home with a partner or children or as a consumer. For some it seems easy, but others view the process of negotiation as a source of conflict to be avoided.

Negotiation is an essential skill for those involved in telephone triage because there are occasions when what a caller wants is not always what is needed or can be provided. Health service staff often find themselves having to act as the interface between competing interests. The health service is a complex, diverse organisation and it would be unrealistic to expect everyone involved in delivering and receiving its services to always agree. Therefore, negotiation skills are very important.

However, the call handler also needs to be able to recognise situations where it is not appropriate to

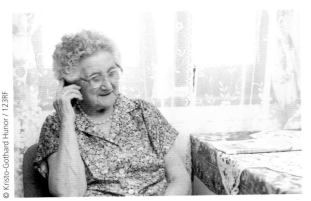

© Kristo-Gothard Hunor / 123RF

Figure 3.3 It may be unrealistic to expect a frail, elderly person who lives alone without access to transport to travel independently to the emergency department

persuade callers to accept our initial advice. It may well be that what you are advising cannot be achieved or carried out by the caller/patient. For example, it may be unrealistic to expect a frail, elderly person who lives alone and has no access to transport to travel independently to the emergency department (Figure 3.3). Conversely, to expect a younger caller who has access to private or public transport to travel may be an entirely realistic point of negotiation.

Where negotiation does occur, it should never become a conflict situation. Negotiation does not mean being domineering or rude, but it does mean being assertive. Assertiveness is about communicating in a way that demonstrates 'respect for me and respect for you'. The basis of good negotiation is forming a good relationship with the caller. Using a polite and friendly approach from the start will help to build the necessary trust and respect. There may be a number of reasons for caller resistance which will be discussed within this section. However, this does not change the way you should handle a call. Being polite and friendly is the best way to build trust and establish an effective rapport.

Understanding the Reasons for Caller Resistance

Understanding the possible reasons for resistance is vital in helping you to decide whether to negotiate and, if so, what approach to take.

Resistance to your advice may be due to a lack of understanding about the service which you are recommending. The NHS is very complex and can be hard to navigate. Research has shown that there is a lack of awareness about NHS services, what they provide and how and when they can be accessed. We should not expect patients to be experts in this. People may know that an alternative service is more appropriate but have experienced difficulty accessing it in the past. It is also human nature when we have a problem to want it dealt with quickly, even if it is not clinically justified.

Anxiety often causes people to respond in ways they would not normally. This can include aggression, silence or rudeness. A patient's anxiety about a symptom may be entirely justified. If someone seems very anxious or insistent that the problem requires a different response from the one you are advising, treat this as a warning sign. It is vital to ask yourself if you may have missed something and if you have listened properly. It may be necessary for you to clarify your understanding of the situation or to seek clinical advice.

Social disadvantage can play a part in a caller resisting your advice, for example, accessing certain services can be difficult without transport or the means to pay for this. Loneliness and isolation can also be factors to consider. Receiving a face-to-face consultation may, in some cases, fulfil needs other than health needs (for instance someone's need for reassurance) or it may reduce a sense of isolation.

Sensitive questioning will often reveal the reason for resistance; this then helps you to decide on the most appropriate approach to take.

Dahlgren and Whitehead's (1991) model of social factors and health outlines the different socioeconomic, cultural and environmental conditions which can affect a person's health.

The Negotiation Process

1. Active Listening

   This is about picking up on the messages being sent, whilst letting the other person know that you have listened. This means listening to the things that are said (the words), how they are said (the emphasis) and the emotions revealed (what is not said).

Active listening requires you to focus on the other person without thinking about your next question or response and without focusing on the environment around you. It requires 100% of your attention. This is about the 'respect for you' element of assertiveness.

Active listening shows you take others seriously but it does not necessarily mean agreeing with their standpoint. Analysis of calls where something has gone wrong shows that there is a dangerous tendency for people to pay less attention once the necessary triage questions have been asked. However, this is often when important information or emotions are 'restated'. Active listening at this point may yield bits of information that mean you need to reassess the situation. Is the patient demanding more attention because they are really seriously ill, or because they've had a bad experience with the health service? Is someone's difficulty understanding simply due a cultural difference, or does it indicate a mental health problem or learning disability? Everyone gets things wrong from time to time. There may be situations where you have missed an important piece of information during the initial assessment; their insistence that your advice is wrong may be justified.

2. Putting your point across

    If you are sure that the outcome you've advised is the right one, this is the time to explain why. Whilst this part of the process does not involve you being stubborn or domineering, it is about you holding on to a sense that what you are trying to do matters and is important. Essentially, it's about the 'respect for me' part of assertiveness.

    You should put your points firmly but in a friendly manner. Remind the caller that you have been listening by using information provided by them to back up your advice, for example, 'You said that Mary hasn't got any other symptoms'. This will help them understand the reasons behind your advice and give them more confidence that it is appropriate.

3. Working towards a 'win–win' solution.

    Once you have put your point, listen carefully to what the caller has to say in response. If they do not want to follow your advice, stop and think about why. Have you been clear in what you were saying? Did you sound confident and believe in what you were advising? Importantly, have you missed something or not given enough emphasis to what the caller told you? Do you need to revisit parts of your assessment?

Once you have understood the caller's response you need to try and move the situation along towards a win–win solution where each party feels their needs are being met.

The reasons for any resistance should determine your actions. You may need to concede to them if the issue is insurmountable, such as a severe mental health problem or communication problem. You may need to reassess the situation if it seems you have missed something. If the problem is due to a lack of knowledge, for instance how to access a certain service, you will need to address this knowledge gap.

If you are not able to negotiate an agreed outcome, make sure you follow your local processes to deal safely with this. If the caller is clearly not going to follow your advice, it is still important to help them form a clear plan of what to do next. Finally, as with any caller, it is essential to end the call making sure they are clear in the knowledge about what to do should they have further concerns. This is essential from a risk management perspective.

Checklist of skills/attitudes needed for effective negotiation

1. Excellent communication

    Unless you are a skilled listener and have an effective way of putting your point across, you are unlikely to be a skilled negotiator.

2. Empathy and sensitivity

    Putting yourself in the caller's shoes may help you understand the reasons for any resistance and help you deal sensitively with this.

3. Checking out beliefs and assumptions

    The process of checking out beliefs and assumptions should help to reduce areas of disagreement as you are more likely to be talking on the same 'wavelength'.

4. Assertiveness

   Remember, this does not mean being domineering. It means communication. This shows respect both for yourself and the other person involved.

5. Keeping it friendly

   It is essential to keep things friendly and avoid a battle of wills. People are far more likely to respond reasonably if you stay friendly.

Summary

Communication is a natural skill that we use on a constant basis. However, the skills of telephone communication are not quite the same as those we use in a face-to-face context. Being a skilled communicator is absolutely at the heart of being a skilled call handler. Being a skilled communicator over the telephone involves many different facets such as active listening, skilled questioning, building rapport, demonstrating warmth and empathy. It also involves overcoming the inevitable barriers and challenges to communication that you will

encounter on a very regular basis. Only when you can overcome barriers can you be sure of providing patients with the advice and care they need.

It is not enough just to read about the skills involved; you also need to practice and reflect on your skills. Nevertheless, understanding what makes communication effective over the telephone is an essential first step in becoming a skilled call handler.

References and Further Reading

Collins Online Dictionary (2017). Available at: www.collinsdictionary.com/dictionary/english/probe (last accessed 21 April 2017).

Corcoran, N. (2013). *Communicating Health: Strategies for Health Promotion.* London: SAGE.

Dahlgren, G. and Whitehead, M. (1991). *Policies and Strategies to Promote Social Equity in Health.* Stockholm, Sweden: Institute for Futures Studies.

HSCIC (2016). *Data on Written Complaints in the NHS.* Available at: http://content.digital.nhs.uk/catalogue/PUB21536/data-writ-comp-nhs-2016-2017-Q1-rep.pdf (last accessed 20 April 2017).

Pilbery, R. and Lethbridge, K. (2016). *Ambulance Care Practice.* Bridgwater: Class Publishing.

Chapter 4: Critical Thinking in Telephone Triage

Learning Objectives

By the end of this chapter you will be able to:
- Define critical thinking
- Explain the need for critical thinking within telephone triage
- Discuss how to form a 'big picture' in order to make effective decisions
- Recognise the impact of biases and assumptions
- Summarise a range of factors that contribute to effective critical thinking.

Introduction

If you make decisions on the basis of inaccurate or incomplete information it is not likely to be an effective decision. This matters enormously within telephone triage, where people's lives can be at stake. The process of collecting the right information and analysing it effectively to make good decisions is called 'critical thinking'. Although critical thinking skills can be used to expose poor reasoning, it is also an essential component in forming cooperative relationships with others.

Using a clinical decision support system (CDSS) does not remove the need for decision making. For example, these are just some of the decisions you might need to make:
- Do I need to talk to the patient?
- Is the caller understanding me?
- Does the information provided by a caller answer the question adequately?
- Do I need to ask the question in front of me, or has the caller already answered it?
- Which route shall I take through the system? (This is, in effect, a string of different decisions.)
- Does this outcome seem right?
- Do I need to clarify anything?
- Does the caller seem likely to follow my advice and what do I need to do about this?

What is Critical Thinking?

Critical thinking is the ability to think clearly and rationally about how to act or what conclusions to come to. Someone with critical thinking skills is able to:
- Identify and understand logical connections between ideas (e.g. a logical connection might be that a person moaning in pain in the background is the patient with pain that is being discussed).
- The next step in critical thinking would be the need to identify your own thought processes (e.g. was the person moaning in pain the patient?). This analysis of your own thought processes and assumptions is a critical way to avoid 'bias' or to come to conclusions based on what might be flawed information (e.g. it could be someone other than the patient moaning in the background!).
- Detect inconsistencies and irregularities (e.g. picking up on the fact that the patient moaning in the background is speaking in full sentences in-between peaks of pain, even though the caller has said they can't).
- Identify, construct and evaluate theories (e.g. 'The patient seems to be talking okay. How can I sensitively put this to the caller to check it out?').
- Identify the relevance and importance of ideas (e.g. What information is important to the assessment? What is less relevant?).
- Solve problems systematically (e.g. if a caller objects to the final outcome of the call, a critical thinker will go through a structured process of explaining the reason for the outcome, establishing why the caller rejects the advice, revisiting parts of the assessment where necessary and possibly referring on to a more senior colleague if there is still an issue).

Listen for Ideas – Not Just Words

Critical thinking is not just about accumulating information; it is analysing and weighing up information, rather than just collecting more and more. Discarding information appropriately is also vital.

One of the most difficult aspects of listening is the ability to link together pieces of information to form a coherent 'picture' of the overall situation. However, with proper concentration this process becomes easier. Sometimes, callers will gradually offer individual pieces of information throughout the call. In these instances, you need to carefully assimilate the information being offered to gauge its relevance to the call. It may help to jot these down as they arise so as not to lose track of them.

Someone with strong critical thinking skills can often take in extra information and sort out the important nuggets without allowing the extraneous information to influence the call. However, as a non-clinician, you may be presented with complex clinical information that requires the skill of someone clinical to interpret it. Therefore your task as a call handler with strong critical thinking skills is to recognise these situations and respond appropriately by getting some clinical support or transferring the call.

Biases and Assumptions

We all have biases and we all make assumptions. For example, in the height of summer you can assume that heavy frosts won't occur so you don't need to sprinkle salt on your path every night! Or to take an example relevant to work, you can assume that someone calling your service with athlete's foot would have mentioned if they were also suffering from severe chest pain. Life would be extremely difficult if we didn't all make sensible assumptions every day. This is a form of critical thinking known as 'inference' whereby you reach logical conclusions based on information assumed to be true. The problem arises if the basis on which you are making such assumptions is biased, faulty or inaccurate.

> ## Time out activity – think about some of the assumptions you have made today
> - What information did you base these assumptions on?
> - What impact did these assumptions have?
> - What might be the likely outcome if any of these assumptions is incorrect?

There is a phenomenon within healthcare known as 'wellness bias': there is an underlying belief that people are more well than they actually are. One early study showed that doctors working in a primary care setting were more inclined to underestimate the extent of a baby's illness than their hospital-based colleagues, as the primary care doctors were more used to working in an environment with a lower rate of serious illness [Perrin and Goodman, 1978].

Analysis of calls where there has been a negative outcome often highlights 'wellness bias'. Anecdotally, this seems to be particularly true in services that might not have been set up primarily to take emergency calls. However, patients/carers don't always know which service they should contact. Therefore, emergency-focused services such as the ambulance service will always need to be able to deal with minor illness and non-emergency-focused services need to be able to deal with life-threatening situations. Your decision support system provides the means to conduct safe assessments in the setting that you work in, but only if you don't manipulate the system to give the outcome you assume to be right, especially if the basis for such assumptions is biased or faulty in some way.

> ## Time out activity – examining bias and assumptions
> Take a moment to think about some of the assumptions you tend to make at work and any biases you hold. You do not need to share this information with anyone else unless you want to, but it is only a useful exercise if you are honest.
> - Consider what assumptions you might make on the basis of the patient's age, gender, social circumstances, accent, profession, language, demeanour, perceived educational status and so on.

- How do these biases influence your thinking?
- How do these biases influence your actions?
- What has contributed to you forming these biases?
- What might be the consequences (good and bad) of these assumptions and biases?
- How can you avoid making assumptions on the basis of faulty, inaccurate or incomplete information?

7. Understand the meaning and impact of the conclusion and outcome you deliver for the patient. This means understanding the 'real world' impact of your advice for each individual patient. You can deliver an outcome which is entirely sound from a clinical perspective, but if the patient can't follow the advice it's of no real benefit to them.

Seven steps to improve your critical thinking

1. Identify the problem clearly. Within telephone triage this involves honing in on the clinical issue of concern, as well as the patient's expectations.
2. Be aware of what perspective you bring to the issue: your experience, knowledge, your worldview (e.g. you might have experienced a similar problem, which may colour how you handle it).
3. Be aware of your biases and potential assumptions (e.g. you might think that certain demographic groups always exaggerate their symptoms which might cause you to take their situation less seriously).
4. Follow a sound decision-making process. Within telephone triage, this means conducting effective assessments involving skilled use of your decision support tools.
5. Ensure you process the right information and don't get misled by irrelevant information. This combines the skills of active listening and effective questioning with the ability to sift through information to find what matters.
6. Understand the basis for your decision making so that you can correct any areas that went wrong. This requires an in-depth understanding of the assessment process and tools so that you can unpick it if a mistake has been made or the caller volunteers additional information that makes a difference.

Summary

To deliver safe and effective outcomes for patients within telephone triage it is vital to have good critical thinking skills. Critical thinking is the ability to think in a clear and rational way about how to act or what conclusions to come to. Deciding these next steps, of what to think or how to act, relies on having the right information. If you make decisions on the basis of inaccurate or incomplete information it is not likely to be an effective decision. This matters enormously within telephone triage, where peoples' lives can be at stake. Critical thinking is a skill that can be developed with practice and experience. It relies on other skills and abilities such as active listening, effective picture building, weighing up information and avoiding making assumptions on the basis of faulty or incomplete information. It also requires you to become aware of any biases you might hold, in order that you can take active steps to 'dismantle' these.

Reference

Perrin, E. and Goodman, H. (1978). Telephone Management of Acute Pediatric Illness, *New England Journal of Medicine,* 298(3): 130–135.

Chapter 5: Legal, Ethical and Professional Considerations

Learning Objectives

By the end of this chapter you will be able to:

- Explain the principles of confidentiality in relation to your role
- Describe what is meant by 'duty of care'
- Explain what is meant by negligence
- State the meaning and rationale for whistleblowing within the NHS
- Explain what is meant by 'duty of candour'
- Describe the concepts of consent and capacity
- Summarise the principles of equality and diversity
- State the risks of inappropriate use of social media and list personal strategies to prevent this
- Describe the call handling role in relation to the provision of information
- Explain the need for professional note-taking
- Summarise the requirements of METHANE in relation to communication during a time of serious incident management.

Introduction

Working within healthcare is an extraordinarily privileged role. As a call handler you will be privy to the most sensitive and private information and will often be dealing with people at their most vulnerable. We all have a right to expect that any healthcare we receive will be given according to appropriate professional standards. These standards may rely on a legal framework, ethical requirements or certain professional requirements that may, for example, be embodied within your contract of employment.

Legal and Ethical Issues for Call Handlers within Telephone Triage

Confidentiality

All staff providing healthcare on behalf of the NHS are bound by a legal duty of confidence to protect personal information they may come into contact with during the course of their work. This is not just a requirement of their contractual responsibilities but also a requirement within the common law duty of confidence and the Data Protection Act 1998. Failure to protect a patient's confidentiality can cause distress for the patient and can also result in legal or disciplinary action for both organisations and individuals [NHS England, 2016].

All healthcare providers should have organisational policies in place about handling patient information. You should be made aware of your own local policy when you receive initial training and preparation for your role.

Within your role as a call handler, you will routinely have access to confidential, patient-identifiable information. This needs to be protected, so you should record, handle and store it in such a way that prevents you from breaching the patient's confidentiality.

Person-identifiable information is anything that contains the means to identify a person, including name, address, postcode, date of birth or NHS number [NHS England, 2016]. Confidential information also includes information that is private and not public knowledge or information that an individual would not expect to be shared [NHS England, 2016].

According to NHS England (2016), some good practice guidelines for protecting confidentiality include:

- Seek consent before sharing information.
- Share only information which is necessary.

- Never give out information to persons who do not 'need to know' in order to provide healthcare. If you are asked to disclose information and you are unsure of whether you should, make sure you refer this to a more senior colleague.

- Treat information about patients as confidential and use it only for the purposes for which it was given.

- Log off or 'lock' computers when leaving your desk.

- If identifiable information needs to be sent via e-mail then you should do so via a secure system.

- When speaking on the phone, check whether you have taken all reasonable steps to ensure you are speaking to the correct person.

- Access only the information that you need.

- If using paper records, make sure they are stored securely.

- Shred any documents or notes that are no longer required.

Time out activity – consider the following scenario

A call to a telephone triage service is received regarding a patient who is closely related to one of the shift leaders. The call raises some safeguarding issues. The call handler who manages the call wants to talk to the shift leader about the details of case because he thinks it might ultimately be helpful for the caller.

Before reading on, take some time to think through what the call handler should do.

The call handler in the case study above should follow all normal processes in managing the call and raise any safeguarding issues in the usual way. It would be a breach of the caller's confidentiality to talk about the call to the shift leader. It would be a very inappropriate thing to do, since this sharing would not be based on any 'need to know'. The caller has a right to expect that their information is kept confidential – they did not call to alert a relative of the issue and have not consented to this information being shared. Take a moment to think about what the possible consequences might be. Would the caller be inclined to make contact again if they could not trust that their information was kept confidential and used appropriately? What might happen if

the shift leader was the perpetrator of any suspected abuse or felt inclined to take personal action in relation to any possible issues?

Care also needs to be taken not to breach confidentiality inadvertently. Never talk about patients/staff in public places or where you can be overheard. Be careful not to leave any records, documents or confidential information unattended. In relation to this, it's important to make sure that computers are locked if you leave your workstation and always ensure that screens are not visible to any visitors in the call centre. Finally, make sure that if you maintain a reflective journal, you do not include any identifiable patient information.

Duty of Care

Duty of care is a civil law concept within the UK and exists to ensure that one party does not allow unreasonable harm or loss to occur to another [Dimond, 2011].

Within the NHS, you owe a duty of care to your patient from the point at which they first make contact with the service. From that point onwards, you must act in a way to prevent harm where a reasonable person could see that harm might occur. If you breach this duty of care and someone suffers as a result, this can lead to the civil wrong of negligence.

Scenario – duty of care

Jason has been with 999 for two years and has become very disillusioned with his job. He frequently works weekends and nights, because it suits his family life. However, this means that he receives a lot of calls regarding alcohol misuse. One night he is handling a call from a young man who is demanding an ambulance and appears to be drunk. The caller slurs his words and is verbally aggressive. Jason puts the caller on mute and remarks to his colleague that he's sick and tired of 'drunks and layabouts' and he's going to end the call. Jason cuts off the caller and carries on with the rest of his shift. The caller is subsequently found unconscious by a relative and an ambulance is sent. It is discovered that the patient is a diabetic in a hypoglycaemic coma.

Jason had made an assumption that the patient's demeanour was due to alcohol, which affected the way he dealt with the call. Jason had a duty of care to the patient, irrespective of the cause of his symptoms.

Remember that one of the fundamental principles of the NHS is to put the patient at the heart of everything it does. Patients are the reasons that the NHS exists and the duty of care should always be uppermost in the mind of all healthcare staff.

Negligence

Negligence occurs when a duty of care is breached and reasonably foreseeable harm occurs as a result. Negligence cases can be pursued through the civil courts for damages. There are four stages necessary for negligence to be proven [Pilbery, 2013]:

- Establish a duty of care
- Establish breach of duty
- Establish harm occurred
- Establish causation.

Let us think about each of these in turn.

Establishing a duty of care is usually straightforward (e.g. once you answer a call to a patient, you owe them a duty of care).

Breach of duty occurs when a reasonably foreseeable consequence of a person's action leads to harm. It can be difficult to decide what is 'reasonably foreseeable': this is a point that the courts may have to decide upon.

A patient must be harmed or suffer a loss for a claim to be successful. For any harm alleged, it must be proved that this was due to the actions or omissions of the practitioner. The definition of harm is very wide and types of harm may include:

- Physical harm
- Emotional distress
- Loss of income or future earnings
- Loss of enjoyment of life.

Causation is the final step in proving negligence. It is not enough for a duty of care to be breached. That has to go on to cause harm and it should be evident that this breach was the cause. Sometimes referred to as the 'but for' principle, it is applied by asking 'But for (the action or omission), would harm have occurred?' If the answer to this is 'Yes', then negligence is not proven. If the answer is 'No', then it is likely that negligence exists.

Time out activity – duty of care

Take a few moments to think about the case study described in the last section.

- Did Jason have a duty of care? Why?
- Did Jason breach a duty of care? How?
- Did the patient suffer harm? What was this?
- Did any breach of a duty of care cause harm?

As soon as they answered the call, the call handler had a duty to provide care for the patient. The harm the patient suffered was possible emotional distress at not being able to summon the help they needed and subsequently becoming unconscious. Whether the call handler was responsible for the harm that occurred would be for a court to decide. However, it is clear that this is one possible conclusion.

Whistleblowing

Improving patient safety relies on staff identifying when they have concerns about the way things are done or when mistakes have been made. An open and transparent culture helps organisations learn from problems and mistakes in order to make the necessary improvements. Whistleblowing is the act of reporting suspected wrongdoing at work. Whistleblowers should be supported and encouraged to speak up, rather than punished for their actions. However, historically whistleblowers have not always been treated fairly by their employers, with instances of bullying and dismissal occurring [Francis, 2015].

Time out activity – whistleblowing

Consider the following scenario. A member of training staff within an organisation is told by their manager, that for a period of six months, they should stop doing written and practical assessments of call handlers during initial training. The trainer objects strenuously to this, pointing out that assessment of trainees is essential to identify learning needs, spot knowledge gaps and assess overall competence and safety. The manager replies saying that they are under enormous pressure to fill vacancies and that 'everyone must pass the course!' The trainer is unsure what to do next.

Spend a few minutes considering the following questions:

- What is the trainer's responsibility in this situation?
- What might be the consequences of the trainer not taking these concerns further?
- What might be the consequences of the trainer taking these concerns further?

Clearly this trainer has a responsibility to act on the concerns they have. Failure to do so may put patients, staff and the organisation at risk.

Reporting concerns properly is important, as it provides protection for the whistleblower, as well as a structured process to follow. Your organisational policy on whistleblowing should outline who to raise a concern with and the appropriate route for escalating it if necessary.

Duty of Candour

Duty of candour is a direct result of the Francis report referred to in the previous section. It places a legal obligation on healthcare providers to inform a patient if they have been harmed by the provision of healthcare and offer an appropriate remedy, regardless of whether a complaint has been made or a question asked. For healthcare organisations, this is a standard of their regulation by the Care Quality Commission [CQC, 2014].

If you believe that the actions you have undertaken have caused a patient harm, or may cause harm at some future point, you should report this immediately in an open and honest manner. Do not wait for a complaint to be received or for a question to be asked before highlighting the issue. Dealing with an issue quickly can sometimes mean that any likely harm can be minimised. Any deliberate failure to observe your duty of candour could be seen as a breach of your duty of care.

Scenario – duty of candour

Consider the following scenario. Ajahn handles a call regarding a young child with abdominal pain, vomiting and confusion. The parent calling seems relatively unconcerned and Ajahn is reassured by this. Ajahn focuses on the abdominal pain and vomiting and following the assessment advises the caller that the child needs to be seen within primary care within the next six hours. The caller accepts this and the call ends.

After the call Ajahn has a niggling feeling that he has missed something. He goes over the call in his mind and realises that he did not pay any attention to the caller's description of the child's confusion. Ajahn reflects that it is not normal and wonders if he was influenced by the caller's calm and unconcerned demeanour. He recalls some critical thinking training he received recently, that focused on 'wellness bias' and the importance of not making assumptions just because of a caller's demeanour.

Ajahn approaches a clinical colleague and discusses his concerns. During the discussion, Ajahn realises that there were other symptoms that he did not pay much attention to, such as slight breathlessness and extreme pallor. The clinician agrees to make contact with the caller to reassess the situation. On doing so, it is discovered that the child is booked into the GP surgery in about six hours' time, but that she is really quite unwell and her parents didn't know what to do. The reassessment carried out determines that the child needs an ambulance.

The child is seen in an emergency department and a diagnosis of sepsis is made. Prompt treatment is given and the child makes a full recovery.

The scenario illustrates the importance of being open and honest if you feel that there may be a risk of patient harm. It also demonstrates the importance of reporting concerns without delay, because it may be possible to prevent such harm occurring or limit the extent of this harm.

Consent and Capacity

Consent and capacity are important concepts for anyone working within healthcare. In the United Kingdom, adult patients with 'mental capacity' must give permission or 'consent' before they are touched or treated.

In order for consent to be valid, there are three criteria that must be met [NHS Choices, 2014]. These are:

- Consent must be given voluntarily. It must be free from pressure exerted by family, friends, professionals, etc.

- Consent must be informed. The patient must understand what course of action is being proposed, what the benefits and significant risks are, what alternatives are available and the consequences of doing nothing.

- The person consenting needs to have the mental capacity to do so. This is usually the patient, but includes someone with parental responsibility in patients less than 18 years of age or a person who has been given a Lasting Power of Attorney or authority by a court to make treatment decisions [DoH, 2009]. Any adult with capacity can register a Lasting Power of Attorney. This means appointing another person to make decisions on their behalf, if they are unable. A Lasting Power of Attorney must be registered with the Office of the Public Guardian and has wide-ranging powers to make decisions in the event of the patient being incapacitated.

As a rule, if your patient is over 18, only they can consent to any intervention. Within telephone triage, this does not mean that you are unable to carry out triage through a third party. However, if the patient is to receive any subsequent treatment as a result of the call, the rules of consent and mental capacity would apply.

Let's think a little bit more about the notion of 'capacity'. In order to consent to treatment, a patient must have the mental capacity to do so voluntarily and in an informed way. Mental capacity is the ability to make a decision. There is no single objective test of this ability, however the requirements for capacity are laid out in The Mental Capacity Act 2005. In a face-to-face setting, healthcare professionals must make decisions and judgements everyday about whether someone has mental capacity. A lack of capacity means that someone is unable to make a specific decision at the time it is required, due to an impairment of, or disturbance in, the functioning of the mind [Dimond, 2011]. It does not matter if this impairment or disturbance is temporary or permanent.

Time out activity – mental capacity

Look back at the case study concerning Hugo on page 14.

When the ambulance crew arrived, they would have had to make a judgment about whether he had the mental capacity to refuse treatment. They would have needed to contact the police. Given his state of mind, it is questionable whether Hugo had mental capacity at the time of his mental health crisis. If he refused care and they felt he lacked mental capacity he could potentially be transported against his wishes to the hospital for appropriate care and treatment.

Mental capacity can be a somewhat fluid state and the concept relates to a specific decision needing to be made at a specific point in time. Hugo may well have lacked mental capacity at the time described, but this is not likely to be a permanent inability to make informed and rational decisions.

Another useful example to explore is in relation to patients with dementia. Some patients may have the capacity to make simple decisions such as purchasing essential items, but they may lack the capacity to make more complex long-term investment decisions.

It is also worth mentioning 'Deprivation of Liberty Safeguards' (DoLS) at this point. DoLS are a way of protecting patients who are necessarily being deprived of their liberty to keep them safe (e.g. patients that lack capacity and are resident in either hospital or care homes [Alzheimer's Society, 2014]). Liberties they are deprived of may include not being allowed to leave their residence when they wish to do so, medication being administered against their will and staff restricting a person's access to family and friends.

As you can see, mental capacity is not a fixed status and does require judgement on the part of professionals. If you are ever in doubt about how to manage someone who seems to lack capacity, you must seek appropriate support.

Equality, Diversity and Discrimination

A focus on equality ensures that organisations work in a way that is fair, so that no community, group or individual is disadvantaged or discriminated against in the delivery of care. Promoting equality should be at the heart of a healthcare organisation's values. [NHS England, 2015].

Before discussing the concepts in more detail, it is helpful to understand the meaning of the terms 'diversity', 'equality', 'inclusion' and 'discrimination'.

- Diversity: this involves recognising and valuing the difference between individuals across groups. Such difference should be seen as 'assets to be valued and affirmed, rather than as problems to be solved' [Thompson, 2006].

- Equality: in its simplest form, this is about being treated fairly. Equality recognises that people are different, but those differences do not mean that a person should be disadvantaged.

- Inclusion: positively striving to meet the needs of different people and taking deliberate action to create environments where everyone feels respected and able to achieve their full potential [NIHR, 2012].

• Discrimination: this occurs when someone treats one person less favourably than they would another, because of a personal characteristic. This is often due to stereotyping.

Considerable health inequalities still exist in our country, so all healthcare professionals have a responsibility to promote equality. The Kings Fund (2015) discusses how men and women from the richest social groups live an average of seven years longer than those from the poorest social class. Issues that are thought to influence health inequalities include:

• Employment
• Education
• Availability and accessibility to healthcare
• Housing.

Working in healthcare, you should be doing all you can to ensure the equitable provision of healthcare to all of your patients and supporting them to overcome health inequalities where they exist. This may be as simple as talking a homeless person through the process of registering with a GP, or using interpreter services for patients who do not speak English, like the call handler did with Rumbi in Chapter Two.

Earlier, in the section on critical thinking, you were encouraged to examine your biases. We all have biases, but the important thing is to be aware of these and not to let them influence your actions. Acting on bias is one of the ways that healthcare staff can inadvertently perpetuate or create inequalities in health.

Time out activity – recognising personal bias

Consider the following scenario. Jade is a call handler. She is a single mother of three children all under the age of six. Jade works full time and has done since her youngest child was four months old. Jade fell pregnant during her first term at university and had to drop out.

The service that Jade works for is based in a large university city and she regularly handles calls from students with various health concerns. Jade handles a call regarding a 21-year-old student who is suffering from severe anxiety and panic attacks which seem to be being triggered by exam pressure. This call is audited by Jade's supervisor. Afterwards Jade is invited to listen to the call as there are some concerns about the way she handled it. On listening, Jade realises that she sounded cold and unconcerned. She seems to robotically move through the questions she needed to ask without injecting any sense of care, compassion or empathy. At the end of the call, it is clear that there is no rapport between Jade and the caller and it is questionable whether he will follow her advice.

Jade cares deeply about the work she does and takes some time to reflect. She realises that she has some resentment about not being able to continue with her university education. Phrases such as 'all students are lazy', 'students do not know how lucky they are' and 'students never appreciate the opportunity they've been given' swirl around in her head.

Jade contemplates whether she has a disdainful attitude to students who seem to be struggling with their time at university. She concludes that she is not providing the best service to certain types of callers. As Jade is a skilled critical thinker, she is able to start questioning her stereotypes and biases through a process of reflection. She realises that she may always harbour some disappointment at her own personal situation, but that it is wrong to let this impact on the quality of care she gives.

Consider the following questions:
• What stereotypes does Jade hold?
• How do these affect Jade's practice?
• Might Jade's handling of the call be considered to be discriminatory?
• How might Jade's management of the call perpetuate or lead to health inequality?

In order to make sense of society and those in it, we naturally group individuals together when they share common characteristics. We may expect people within the group to act in similar ways or to have similar responses to the same situations. This process is called stereotyping [Judd, 1993] and it was clearly something that Jade was doing.

Using these stereotypes is a natural process as it allows us to 'shortcut' our thinking. Often, stereotypes are inaccurate. Making such shortcuts in healthcare can be dangerous if it means we alter our behaviour, particularly if our assumptions are faulty in some way. It is also harmful if it means we treat some groups in society less favourably.

It's clear to see how Jade's life experiences have contributed to the formation of certain stereotypes and biases. If she was able to prevent her behaviour being affected by these stereotypes, then she would be able to avoid being biased in her approach.

Sometimes, however, we are not even aware of the stereotypes we use and may act almost as though we are on 'auto-pilot'. Fortunately, the issue was picked up by a manager and Jade was given the opportunity to reflect on her thinking to prevent a similar situation happening again.

> ## Time out activity – stereotyping
> - What stereotypes have you become aware of in colleagues around you?
> - What impact might these have had?
> - What stereotypes do you hold?
> - What impact might these have on your call handling role?
> - What do you need to do to avoid acting on these stereotypes?

During the course of your call handling role, you may observe signs of discrimination in practice. This should be challenged as it can have an adverse impact on patient care and can be responsible for the perpetuation of health inequalities. If discrimination is allowed to continue unchallenged it can become embedded in everyday practice and organisational culture.

Challenging discrimination can be difficult, and if not done in an appropriate way it can lead to conflict. Each situation will be unique. However, in general it can be helpful to promote discussion, rather than telling someone they have got it wrong. During discussion people will often realise that their thinking is faulty in some way. Staying non-critical and non-judgemental is likely to encourage an environment where people feel safe to discuss difficult and complex issues. If you feel you are not able to challenge discrimination directly, make sure you get some guidance and support from someone more senior within your organisation.

Professional Issues for Call Handlers within Telephone Triage

Social Media

Social media is a term used for interactive online media that allow people to communicate instantly with each other, or share information, knowledge, opinions and interests in a public forum. Social media includes the following:

- Social networking sites (e.g. Facebook and LinkedIn)
- Micro-blogging sites (e.g. Twitter)
- Blogs and personal websites
- Messaging boards
- Photo and video content sharing sites (e.g. YouTube, Pinterest and Flickr).

In recent years, the popularity of social media has grown rapidly, but many healthcare workers have found themselves in trouble because of activity on their own personal social media accounts. Some registered professionals such as nurses and paramedics have even been removed from their professional registers for inappropriate use of social media.

Social media makes it possible to share information on a global basis quickly and easily and what you think might be private, often is not.

Of course, some things are obvious in relation to social media. Your legal and ethical duty to safeguard patients' confidentiality applies equally to the internet as to other media. It would also be inappropriate to post informal, personal or derogatory comments about colleagues or your employer. Even if you do not name people or organisations, it is often very easy to work out who comments apply to by a process of elimination. Remember, when you post comments it is often not just your friends and contacts that see them, but their friends and contacts too. When posting on social media you should assume it is in the public domain. Even if something is initially shared with a limited group of followers or friends, there is the potential for it to be copied and shared or published elsewhere. It is important to consider carefully before publishing anything, and work on the basis that anything written or posted could be shared more widely without your knowledge or permission.

You are, of course, entitled to have a private life, but social media can blur the boundaries between personal and work life. It is important that you understand your employment contract and associated policies and how your actions relate to these. For example, would you think it is appropriate to be pictured in your work uniform drinking alcohol? There is a strong possibility that your organisation forbids this in order to uphold a positive reputation and image in the public eye. In any event, what message would such a picture

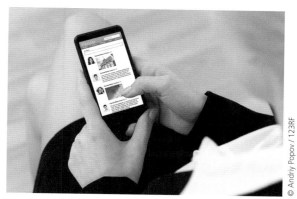

© Andriy Popov / 123RF

Figure 5.1 Posting information directly relating to work-related activity also presents a potential risk, even if your comments are innocent and well intended.

give about the importance and responsibility of your role. This is just an example, but whenever you wear your organisation's uniform you are essentially representing it.

Of course, not everyone drinks alcohol, but let's continue to use this as an example. Most people would find it reasonable and acceptable to see a picture of you with friends and family behaving sensibly around a table with alcohol in the picture. However, a picture of you participating in any behaviour that could be associated with more inappropriate actions and consequences may not feel so acceptable to people who might need to access your care at some point.

It is perhaps easy to adopt an attitude of 'well that's their problem' if someone takes exception to something you've posted that either refers to work or shows you in a potentially negative light. However, as a member of the health service it is important to understand that you serve the public; as such you are required to uphold appropriate standards which do not bring either the health service or your organisation into disrepute.

Posting information directly concerning work-related activity also presents a potential risk, even if your comments are innocent and well intended (Figure 5.1).

Let's consider some examples:

- How could the post in Figure 5.2 be perceived by others?
- Would a caller to 999 expect the person helping them to be *excited* at a time of distress?

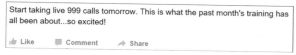

Start taking live 999 calls tomorrow. This is what the past month's training has all been about...so excited!

👍 Like 💬 Comment ➔ Share

Figure 5.2 Social media post 1

Glad the exams weren't today....I would've failed for sure. Definitely having a 'thick' day.

Figure 5.3 Social media post 2

- Would a caller to 999 feel confident that if they called 999 tomorrow an experienced person will answer their call?

Figure 5.3 might seem quite innocent but, coupled with the knowledge that the person works in an organisation such as 999 or 111, it may create negative perceptions such as:

- 'You can't have a "thick" day … you should be working to an excellent standard every day!'
- 'How do I know you weren't just having a 'lucky' day when you did pass your exams?'
- 'If I call and you answer how confident am I in your ability?'
- 'What sort of organisation employs people that can have "thick" days when you deal with people's lives?'

What kind of impression might this post in Figure 5.4 create? Is there a chance that some people may take the following views?

- 'If I call 111 or 999 will I be speaking to a novice?'
- 'Are 111 or 999 call handlers let loose after training? What does that mean?'

This post had also tagged several colleagues, meaning that those tagged are perhaps unwittingly sharing information they have neither created nor consented to. Although you may feel you know your own friends and contacts and are therefore well placed to predict their conclusions about your posts, the same cannot be said of your friends' friends and contacts.

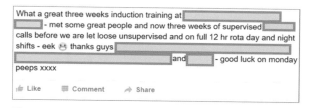

What a great three weeks induction training at ☐☐☐ - met some great people and now three weeks of supervised ☐☐☐ calls before we are let loose unsupervised and on full 12 hr rota day and night shifts - eek 😬 thanks guys ☐☐☐☐☐☐ and ☐☐☐ - good luck on monday peeps xxxx

👍 Like 💬 Comment ➔ Share

Figure 5.4 Social media post 3

Time out activity – reflecting on social media use

- Are there any posts that you may have made that in hindsight you might regret?
- Have you ever commented on an awful shift? How much confidence would that give to a potential user of your service?
- Do you need to review your social media accounts and delete any posts?
- Do you need to 'untag' yourself from posts made by others?

As you may be aware, it has also been known for undercover reporters to target staff who work in NHS trusts and partnership organisations with the sole purpose of finding out information about the NHS and how services are delivered, organised and managed. Make sure you know who you are befriending on social media and ensure you are fully up to date with your employer's social media policy. Take sensible steps to avoid unwittingly putting your employment at risk by not divulging patient-related or confidential information and not making comments about other people in your workplace that could be construed as libellous, bullying or harassment. It may also include political statements that may be perceived to be made in your employer's name.

When used in a positive, deliberate and sensible manner, social media can be an excellent way of maintaining contact with friends and colleagues. However, it is important to make sure that you think carefully about how you portray yourself, your colleagues, your organisation and the NHS as part of your social media activity.

Tips for sensible social media use

- If you would not say something aloud in a public place, do not post it online.
- Ensure you get your facts right.
- Never post information which might be considered inciting, defaming, bullying, or illegal.
- Think about how different people might read your post; if in doubt, do not post.
- Review your privacy settings regularly. Social media sites cannot guarantee confidentiality.
- Remember that once information is online, it can be difficult to remove it.
- Think carefully before tagging other people.

- Take care when sharing or retweeting others' posts as it may be seen as an endorsement of their views.
- Never befriend service users.
- Scrutinise friend requests carefully:
  o Do you really know them?
  o If it is a friend of a friend, check their profiles to see if they seem genuine.
  o Do not accept friends just to increase the number of people you are friends with.

Your Role and the Provision of Information

Information is at the heart of what you do. Your role revolves around the collection of patient-related material, the provision of information to patients, the recording of information collected and given and the transfer of this information to others to enable consistent seamless care. Information is vital in enabling the patient to access the care they need. You are often at the beginning of this chain of information and you have a vital part to play.

Understanding who will use your information is important, because it ensures that you produce information which is useful and relevant.

As we discussed in Chapter Two, the care that you provide can impact on a significant number of other people and organisations. Different people and organisations require different information and will use it in different ways.

How Do You Provide Information?

As a general rule, the information you provide will be both written and verbal. Verbal communication with patients was discussed at length in Chapter Three. Let us have a think about written information within the context of your role.

During the triage process, you will rely heavily on the clinical decision support system (CDSS) in use within your organisation. This will help ensure you ask appropriate questions, the answers to which will likely be recorded automatically into a call log/record. However, there will be times when you have to add extra information in the form of free text to enhance or supplement this information.

You must remember that the record of the call and the audio recording of the interaction form a legal record of the care and advice given to the patient. In the event of a complaint or serious adverse event being reported, the record would need to be reviewed by others including managers within your service. If there is a very serious event, it may be requested by legal representatives, a coroner or the police. The patient is also entitled to access their medical records and this includes records of any telephone consultation. This is not intended to scare you, but merely to reinforce the fact that telephone triage records have the same legal status as any other patient record; as such, you must take care to ensure that they are of an appropriate professional standard.

With most computerised systems it is not possible to delete an entry once it has been saved. Care must be taken to ensure that anyone else using your information can do so efficiently and safely. A good example of this would be in relation to the demographic details you need to take; this may be important if an ambulance crew had to be dispatched.

Note Taking

Whatever your workplace environment, it is likely that as someone involved in telephone triage your main work tools will be a computer, telephone and perhaps other technology-based equipment.

Professional documentation should be:

- Clear – the whole call record should be easy to understand.
- Accurate – the whole call record, including any supplementary notes, should accurately reflect what occurred.
- Concise – supplementary notes should only contain as much detail as is necessary and should only be added when required.
- Adequate – all information recorded, whilst being concise, should contain all essential details and information.
- Without abbreviations or diagnosis – abbreviations should be avoided (apart from those agreed by your organisation) as these can be interpreted in different ways.

Organisations responsible for the delivery of telephone triage must have resilience systems in place in the event of a technology failure. It is important that you are aware of how these operate.

There may be aspects of your role that require you to produce handwritten notes and documents. This may be associated with the resilience tools just referred to, or as another part of your role. Handwritten notes may be needed in the following situations:

- The intended message recipient is unavailable for some reason.
- A call is connected to your telephone extension in error. In this situation you should act professionally and accept responsibility for managing the call in a manner that is commensurate with your training and abilities. Explain if you are unable to manage the call and need to seek assistance from someone else.

Message or memo taking can seem like common sense and indeed it probably is. But getting the basics right is important because when you work in a healthcare setting, the information that needs to be transferred is often very important, detailed or time critical.

Top tips for message/memo taking

- Write clearly
  - Use capital letters if necessary.
  - Any misunderstanding caused by your handwriting may be blamed on you.
- Include the full name of the intended recipient
- Include the full name of the message originator
- Include a contact number for the message originator
  - Include any extension numbers.
  - Repeat this back to the message originator to ensure you have copied it down correctly.
- Record the date that the message was received
  - The recipient may not necessarily read your message on the same day you write it.
- Record the time the message was received
  - This helps the recipient in case they have actually been in communication with the originator since you wrote the message.
- Always add your name so the recipient knows you have written the note
  - Include your full name – there may be others in your place of work who share your first name.
  - Include your contact telephone number – this helps if there are others in your place of work that share you surname too.
- Annotate the note with the exact message intended for the recipient

- Repeat the message back to the originator – this allows for any misunderstanding to be identified and corrected.
- Leave your message in the correct place
  - Use a location your recipient will look at on return to their desk.
  - Consider the need for confidentiality.
  - Have you got the right person's desk?
  - Consider sending a separate alert (e.g. email) to the recipient to let them know there is a written note for their attention.
- Follow up afterwards and check whether the recipient received the message.
- If memo taking is a normal part of your role, obtain a memo pad with a printed format to ensure you include all relevant information.

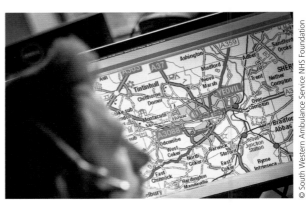

Figure 5.5 All handlers working within a 999 setting may receive incident reports based on METHANE structure

Major Incidents – METHANE

Effective communication is clearly essential when an organisation is responding to a large-scale incident. If you work within an ambulance service, there is a chance you could become involved in this. In the past these types of incidents have included aircraft accidents, multiple vehicle road traffic accidents, terrorist attacks and spree killings. When these kinds of events occur, effective and efficient communication between services is clearly essential to ensure an appropriate and coordinated response.

To enable this, all emergency services use the same digital radio system. To minimise the potential for miscommunication, a single method of information sharing is used. This is based on the mnemonic METHANE which is set out below:

M Major Incident declared? (including date and time of declaration)

E Exact location (geographic area of incident)

T Type of incident (flooding/fire/utility failure/ disease outbreak, etc.)

H Hazards (present or suspected)

A Access (routes that are safe to use, any inaccessible routes)

N Number of casualties (including type and severity)

E Emergency services (present and those required)

Call handlers working within a 999 setting may receive incident reports based on this structure, but it is not inconceivable that non-emergency control rooms may be used as part of a wider response to any major incident affecting public health.

Summary

Anyone working within healthcare is required to uphold certain standards in relation to the legal, ethical and professional management of patients, their information and the way we conduct ourselves. Delivering healthcare often involves being privy to incredibly sensitive information about the most intimate areas of peoples' lives, and we are often dealing with people who are vulnerable, in pain, suffering or distressed in some way. Patients are entitled to expect that those delivering their care do so with a high degree of professionalism, with due regard for all relevant legal and ethical standards.

Useful Links

NHS Employers (2014). *New to the NHS? Your guide to using social media in the NHS*. Available at: www.nhsemployers.org/~/media/Employers/Publications/NOVEMBER%20Your%20guide%20to%20using%20social%20media%20in%20the%20NHS.pdf (last accessed: 4 June 2018).

NHS Employers (2016). *Social Media Guidelines and Tools*. www.nhsemployers.org/your-workforce/need-to-know/social-media-and-the-nhs/social-media-guidelines

References and Further Reading

Material in this chapter has been reproduced from: Richard Pilbery and Kris Lethbridge, *Ambulance Care Practice*, Bridgwater: Class Publishing (2016), with kind permission from the authors.

Alzheimer's Society (2014). *Deprivation of Liberty Safeguards (DoLS): 2015*. Available at: https://www.alzheimers.org.uk/site/scripts/documents_info.php?documentID=1327 (Accessed 10 November 2015).

Department of Health (2009). *Reference Guide to Consent for Examination or Treatment*. Available at: https://www.gov.uk/government/publications/reference-guide-toconsent-for-examination-or-treatment-second-edition (Accessed 5 January 2015).

Dimond, B. (2011). *Legal Aspects of Nursing*, 6th edn. Harlow: Pearson.

Judd, C. and Park, B. (1993). Definition and assessment of accuracy in social stereotypes. *Psychological Review*, 100(1), 109–128.

NIHR (2012). *Diversity and inclusion: what's it about and why is it important for public involvement in research?* Available at: http://www.invo.org.uk/wp-content/uploads/2012/10/involvediversityandinclusionoct2012.pdf (Accessed 11 January 2015).

NHS Choices (2014). *Consent to Treatment*. Available at: http://www.nhs.uk/conditions/consent-to-treatment/pages/introduction.aspx (Accessed 10 November 2015).

NHS England (2015). *Equality and diversity*. Available at: http://www.england.nhs.uk/about/equality/ (Accessed 11 January 2015).

NHS England (2016). Confidentiality Policy. Available at: www.england.nhs.uk/wp-content/uploads/2016/12/confidentiality-policy-v3-1.pdf (last accessed 21 April 2017).

Pilbery, R. Caroline, N.L., American Academy of Orthopaedic Surgeons et al. (2013). *Nancy Caroline's Emergency Care in the Streets*. UK 7th ed. Burlington: Jones and Bartlett Learning.

Pilbery, R. and Lethbridge, K. (2016). *Ambulance Care Practice*. Bridgwater: Class Publishing.

The King's Fund (2015). *Life Expectancy*. Available at: http://www.kingsfund.org.uk/time-to-think-differently/trends/demography/life-expectancy (Accessed 10 November 2015).

Thompson, N (2006). *Anti-Discriminatory Practice: Equality, Diversity and Social Justice*. 4th ed. Basingstoke: Palgrave Macmillan.

Chapter 6: **Safeguarding**

Learning Objectives

By the end of this chapter you will be able to:

- Define the term 'safeguarding'
- Explain the main categories of abuse
- Describe who is susceptible to abuse
- Define safeguarding in relation to children and vulnerable adults
- Discuss the role of safeguarding within telephone triage
- Apply learning from previous safeguarding cases to telephone triage
- Recognise the impact of culture on recognising safeguarding issues
- Summarise a range of other safeguarding issues such as cyber bullying, modern slavery, financial abuse, female genital mutilation and radicalisation
- Explain the importance of reporting concerns and how to gain consent.

Introduction

All healthcare staff have a responsibility to report any incident where there are grounds to suggest that a vulnerable adult or child is at risk of suffering abuse, or where there are concerns about an individual's circumstances.

As a call handler, it is vital to understand who may be vulnerable and to understand the forms of abuse that can take place in order to identify any patients being harmed, abused or neglected. Both adults and children can be vulnerable to abuse. In safeguarding terms an adult is classed by the Care Act 2014 as a person aged 18 years or over and a child is someone under the age of 18.

Time out activity – what is safeguarding?

Before reading on, spend a few minutes reflecting on what safeguarding means to you.

Safeguarding means protecting people's health, wellbeing and human rights, and enabling them to live free from harm, abuse and neglect [CQC, 2015].

What is Abuse?

Abuse is any action by someone that causes significant harm to another person. It can be physical, sexual or emotional, but can also be a lack of love, care and attention. It is never normal or okay. It is a violation of an individual's human and civil rights by (an)other person(s) and must be taken seriously when suspected.

Incidents of abuse may be single acts or multiple incidents, and can affect one or more individuals. It is important to treat all incidents seriously as this could identify patterns of harm or abuse that may be occurring. Effective sharing of information between professional and local agencies is essential for effective identification, assessment and service provision [Gov.uk, 2015].

The four main types of abuse common to both adults and children are [DfE, 2015; DoH, 2011]

- Physical abuse. Examples include: hitting, slapping, burning, poisoning, pushing, and misuse of medication, restraint or inappropriate physical sanctions.

- Psychological/emotional abuse. Examples include: threats of harm or abandonment, deprivation of contact, humiliation, blaming, controlling, intimidation, coercion, harassment, verbal abuse, cyber bullying, isolation or unreasonable and unjustified withdrawal of services or supportive networks.

- Sexual abuse. Examples include: rape, sexual assault, indecent exposure, sexual harassment, inappropriate looking or touching, sexual teasing or innuendo, sexual photography, subjection to pornography or witnessing sexual acts.

- Neglect. Examples include: ignoring medical, emotional or physical care needs, failure to provide access to appropriate health, care and support or educational services, the withholding of the necessities of life, such as medication, adequate nutrition and heating.

All healthcare organisations must have safeguarding policies and procedures in place. This includes ensuring that all staff receive relevant training. Make sure you understand these policies and procedures as safeguarding is a vital part of your role.

Consent from adults should always be sought with the exception of where:

- This would increase the risk to others
- There is legal restriction or overriding public interest
- There is life-threatening risk to the patient who is unreasonably withholding consent
- The patient lacks capacity.

Who is Susceptible to Abuse?

All children are vulnerable to abuse, but those who may be more so include those in the following situations [NICE, 2009]:

- Parental or carer drug or alcohol misuse
- Parental or carer mental health problems
- Intra-familial violence or history of violent offending
- Previous child maltreatment in members of the family
- Known maltreatment of an animal by the carer or parent
- Vulnerable and unsupported parents or carers
- Pre-existing disability in the child.

People are considered to be vulnerable when they are at a greater than normal risk of abuse. For vulnerable adults, this can include [NHS Choices, 2015]:

- Those with learning difficulties
- Older people who are isolated
- Those with memory problems
- Those who are dependent on others for support
- Those whose carer is addicted to alcohol or drugs
- Those who live with a carer.

Safeguarding Children

Child abuse is any action by another person – adult or child – that causes significant harm to a child. The National Society for the Prevention of Cruelty to Children (NSPCC) estimates that over half a million children are abused in the UK each year. A child is anyone under the age of 18.

Safeguarding children is defined under the Children Act 2004 as:

- Promoting the welfare of children
- Protecting children from maltreatment through abuse or neglect
- Ensuring children grow up in circumstances consistent with the provision of safe and effective care that enables them to have optimum life chances and enter adulthood successfully.

Safeguarding Vulnerable Adults

Vulnerable adults may be abused by a wide range of people, including: relatives and friends, professional staff, paid care workers, volunteers, other service users, neighbours and those who deliberately target and exploit the vulnerable [DoH, 2000].

Abuse can occur anywhere such as in the home, in a care setting or even a public place. Abusers can be skilled at explaining away injuries or unusual behaviour and making healthcare staff feel relaxed about the situation they find. As a call handler, you may be the first person they have contacted for help so if you identify any concerns you must report them.

According to the Care Act, safeguarding adults includes:

- Protecting their right to live in safety, free from abuse and neglect
- People and organisations working together to prevent the risk of abuse or neglect, and to stop them from happening
- Making sure people's wellbeing is promoted, taking their views, wishes, feelings and beliefs into account.

A principle of the Care Act 2014 is empowerment. This means personalisation with informed consent. The patient should think 'I am asked what I want as a result of the referral'.

Safeguarding and Telephone Triage

Telephone triage services handle millions of calls a year. Therefore, there is tremendous potential to pick up concerns about child protection and vulnerable adults.

Active listening is one of the most important skills in picking up potential causes for concern. As we discussed in Chapter Three, listening involves listening both to the words used as well as any background noises to assess if what we are hearing is a concern that we need to share with other agencies. You must also listen to your 'gut instinct'. If something does not sound right, make sure you get some advice from a more senior colleague about what to do.

There are no hard and fast rules about the things that should raise your concern in relation to safeguarding, but the NSPCC (2017b) highlights the factors below as being of potential concern. This is not an exhaustive list and you are encouraged to find out more, in addition to making sure that you have received safeguarding training provided by your employer.

These are some examples of issues reported over the telephone that might give rise to safeguarding concerns:
- Bruising in a child that is not yet mobile
- Unusual patterns of bruising such as on soft, fleshy parts of the body or hand/finger print bruising
- Repeated injuries
- Injuries caused by a lack of supervision
- Faltering weight growth and slow development in small children
- Bed-wetting or soiling
- Signs of early sexualisation or promiscuity
- Anal or vaginal soreness, unusual genital discharge or symptoms of a sexually transmitted infection
- Underage pregnancy
- Extensive dental decay which can be a sign of neglect
- A changing or unconvincing story in relation to an injury, or the possibility that injuries are being covered up
- Changes in behaviour and mood
- Changes in eating habits
- Repeated absence from work or school
- Misuse of alcohol or drug use
- Signs of self-neglect
- Self-harm
- Missed medical appointments
- Signs and symptoms of possible skin infections or rashes.

Safeguarding may not be an underlying cause for these issues, but the presence of any concerning signs should always be taken seriously.

Time out activity – consider the following case study

A man calls your service regarding his four-year-old daughter. He explains that he has custody of his daughter who has recently returned home from a weekend visit to her mum's. He goes on to explain that his daughter has just been to the toilet and started to cry whilst urinating. She told her dad that it 'really hurts down below' when she has a wee. When dad checked he noticed a small amount of brownish blood in his daughter's underwear. From what little he was able to observe, her genital area also looked very red. His daughter stated she doesn't know if she hurt herself while she had been away.

What would you do as the call handler managing this call?

Remember, you are an important link in the chain of information gathering that occurs within the health service. If you have information that makes you question whether there is a safeguarding issue, you MUST pass it on.

There could be a perfectly rational explanation for these symptoms. However, vaginal bleeding and soreness in a child this young should not be ignored. By reporting this incident using the appropriate procedures set out by your organisation you are not definitively stating that you believe that a child has been abused in any way. Merely that you have heard something during a call that gives you cause for concern and requires further investigation to rule out abuse as a cause. Failure to report any concerns you may have could mean that important information is not considered and vital pieces of the 'jigsaw' could be missing if this child had been a victim of abuse. Research and repeated enquiries into cases of abuse consistently uncover a reluctance of healthcare staff to record and pass on their concerns appropriately.

Any potential safeguarding incident will need to be investigated further, so accurate documentation of the information you pick up is essential. Remember, you are a vital link in the information chain. Accurate recording of the WHOLE incident by everyone involved allows a greater understanding of that situation to be gained. There have been cases reported anecdotally whereby a call handler is given one explanation of how a vulnerable person came to have certain symptoms or injuries and the attending healthcare professional is offered another. Call handlers may also hear additional information in the background during a call that an attending healthcare professional will have no knowledge of if it is not recorded and reported appropriately. An example of this could be crying or threatening language.

Learning from Previous Child Abuse Cases

The vast majority of abuse and neglect happens behind closed doors and rarely reaches the attention of the public. However, over recent years there have been a number of notable cases. One of these tragic cases was that of Baby P.

In August 2007 Baby P was found dead in his cot after nearly a year of continued abuse. The 17-month-old had sustained over 50 injuries over an eight-month period. He had repeatedly been seen or had been in contact with a number of healthcare professionals and Children's Services. An ambulance was called for Baby P on 2 August 2007 and resuscitation attempts were made. Unfortunately, Baby P had swallowed a tooth after being punched and did not survive. Other injuries included a broken back and ribs, mutilated finger tips and missing finger nails.

Another tragic case is that of Victoria Climbie. Victoria was an eight-year-old girl who was tortured and murdered by her guardian in 2000. Victoria's case is another example of health and social care professionals failing to act appropriately on concerns, and failing to share these concerns across professional and organizational boundaries.

What Can We Learn From This as a Call Handler?

On a number of occasions Baby P was reported to have bruises, swellings and scratches. Bruising is one of the most common manifestations of physical abuse. It is difficult for a child to bruise until they are mobile, but once they are, bruises are a common injury. It follows, then, that bruises in a baby who is not yet mobile should be regarded as unusual [NSPCC, 2012]. A useful reminder is:

'If they can't cruise they shouldn't bruise.'

Knees and shins are common areas for children to bruise; most accidental bruises are seen on bony areas, often on the front of the body. A bump to the head is another common injury in children

who are learning to walk and run. These sorts of injuries generally mark the forehead, nose, centre of the chin or back of the head [NSPCC, 2012].

Bruises on certain parts of the body should give rise to more suspicion. This includes bruises on softer parts of the body such as the ears, neck, buttocks, back and abdomen. Other common features to listen out for are bruising to the forearm, upper arm, back of legs, hands or feet. This can be a sign of a child defending themselves from abuse. These types of bruising may be described to you over the phone and should not be ignored. Clusters of bruising or bruising in the shape of a hand or fingers are clearly a cause for concern, but it is unlikely you will be able to establish such details over the telephone [NSPCC, 2012].

Any bruising needs to be taken into consideration alongside other factors such as the child's developmental stage and medical/social history. This can be done more effectively by someone who can see the individual, but it is important to gather as much information as you can to pass on [NSPCC, 2012].

Learning from Previous Vulnerable Adult Cases

Steven Hoskins, a 38-year-old man with learning disabilities, lived alone. He was tortured and murdered in 2006. Steven had made numerous calls to a number of agencies. He had catastrophic injuries from a fall of more than 30 metres. The post mortem showed that he also had cigarette burns as well as bruises to the neck.

Steven had been taken to the emergency department on a few occasions with chest pains, head injuries, and injuries suffered from being assaulted or inflicting self-harm. He had also had a number of consultations with GP services.

In summary, the serious case review stated that 'all serious case review contributors could have been potential rescuers, but every part of the service had significant failures in this role'. The lack of information sharing and partnership working was severely criticised by the case reviewers.

What Can We Learn From This as a Call Handler?

When a patient describes symptoms of assault or self-harm, your active listening skills are key in identifying if there is any cause for further concern.

Questions that you need to explore might include:

- How did they sustain the injury?
- Who assaulted them?
- What were the circumstances?

Probing effectively is an important skill, as well as listening carefully to the responses and any background clues. Having the confidence to report your concerns is vital as well as an excellent understanding of the processes involved in such reporting.

Culture and Society

We live in a rich and diverse culture within the UK and there are cultural variations in the way families lives their lives. Published case reviews have highlighted that there is often a lack of knowledge about specific cultures and that this can lead to a lack of confidence in reporting or recognising abuse. As a call handler it is not your role to definitively determine whether abuse has happened, merely to pass on any concerns about safeguarding. Whilst always trying to be respectful of cultural diversity, your overriding responsibility in relation to ANY safeguarding concern is to report it appropriately.

Other Safeguarding Issues

There are a range of other, less common but equally troubling safeguarding issues which you may encounter within your role. Understanding these and having some awareness of their existence is the first step in being able to identify concerns. The next vital step is to report these concerns using your safeguarding procedures.

Cyber Bullying

This is a form of abuse that is becoming more and more common. It affects many children and adults and takes place via social media, messaging apps and other online forums. In a survey carried out by Bullying UK, 56% of young people said they have seen others bullied online. This could be in the form of harassment, stalking and/or exclusion. Cyber bullying can make people feel alone, overwhelmed or ashamed. They may have low self-esteem, withdraw from spending time with family and prefer to be on their own. There may

be a change to their personality in that they feel depressed, angry or upset. Some may resort to self-harm or attempt suicide.

Modern Slavery

This is the illegal exploitation of people for personal or commercial gain. It encompasses slavery, human trafficking, forced labour and domestic servitude. Victims are deceived or coerced into a situation and feel unable to leave. Since 2013, there has been a 34% increase in cases of modern slavery.

Financial Abuse

This includes theft, fraud, internet scamming, coercion in relation to an adult's financial affairs or arrangements (including in connection with wills, property, inheritance or financial transactions or the misuse or misappropriation of property, possessions or benefits).

Female Genital Mutilation (FGM)

This is a procedure where the female genitals are cut, injured or changed, but where there is no medical reason for this to be done [DoH, 2016]. The victims are generally girls between infancy and 15 years of age. FGM is performed on a child who is unable to resist or give informed consent and is illegal in the UK. It constitutes child abuse and causes life-long physical, psychological and sexual harm. Symptoms can include constant pain, pain and or difficulty having sex, repeated infections, bleeding, depression and problems passing urine. Factors to listen out for:

- The child is from a cultural background known to practice FGM. Communities that perform FGM are found in many parts of Africa, the Middle East and Asia.
- The child may have been out of the country for a prolonged period of time and/or may say they have had a special procedure.
- They may suffer bladder or menstrual problems.

Counter Terrorism and Anti-Radicalisation

It is a sad fact that terrorism is a problem of our modern society. Radicalisation is defined as the process by which a person comes to support terrorism and forms of extremism leading to terrorism [Home Affairs Committee, 2012].

The government introduced PREVENT as part of their strategy to tackle the problem of people becoming 'radicalised'.

The overall aim of PREVENT is to stop people from becoming terrorists or supporting terrorism. The strategy is wide ranging, covering all forms of terrorism including far-right extremism.

As a healthcare worker, there is a possibility that you may come into contact with individuals who either have been or who are vulnerable to being radicalised. It is important to understand your role and responsibilities under the PREVENT strategy. Remember, this could relate to your colleagues and your callers. Radicalisation usually takes place over time rather than consisting of a one-off event, so intervention to stop the process is possible.

Key points on the recognition and management of those demonstrating extremist views

- Recognise those that are more at risk. The main risk factor for becoming radicalised is vulnerability of some sort. This is a broad description but might include, for example, someone with a learning disability, people who feel socially isolated, younger people, those experiencing an identity crisis of some kind or someone with a belief that their culture is under threat.
- Recognise extremist views in those you interact with. This might be evident through an extreme reaction to certain events or descriptions from friends or family of a gradual or sudden change in beliefs and values
- Do not investigate – this is not your role. Instead you should pass on your concerns to your nominated organisation lead as soon as you become concerned. In most cases this will be the person responsible for safeguarding, but, if in doubt, make sure you ask your manager.

Reporting Concerns and Gaining Consent

All organisations within the healthcare system should have a safeguarding lead and their own referrals process. You should receive specific safeguarding training relevant to your role from your own organisation.

As we have already discussed, it is important to share information regarding any safeguarding concerns you have in relation to vulnerable adults or children.

When considering whether to make a safeguarding referral, it is important that you try to seek the consent of the individual concerned wherever possible. Consent can be overridden in the interest of safety. If you feel that it could potentially make the situation worse or put a patient at further risk, then you must document why the decision to override consent has been taken. This is really important as the agency receiving the referral will need to know whether consent was sought, and if not, the reason for not seeking consent. When discussing consent you should not make any promises that you cannot keep, for example, promising that a specific service will be provided for the caller.

Make sure you are clear about the issue of consent, and if necessary, get some guidance from your safeguarding lead about how this applies to your work setting. It can help to have some scripts that can be used with minor adaptations when you want to talk to callers about passing on safeguarding concerns.

When submitting a referral the information needs to be thorough, concise, timely and factual. Do not give personal opinions. Try to recall word-for-word what was said. You should report all concerns, however small they may seem, as this could be significant in the context of longer-term abuse that is taking place. Remember that you may only have one part of the jigsaw. You may hold vital information that helps to put the pieces of the jigsaw together and enable a child or vulnerable adult to be protected from harm.

This book is not a detailed resource on the subject of safeguarding; it is essential that you receive training and guidance from your own organisation on the subject.

Remember that you work as part of a team. If you are ever in any doubt as to whether to make a referral, make sure you seek advice from a clinical member of staff, a manager or your safeguarding lead.

Safeguarding Scenarios

Scenario 1

A six-week-old baby has fallen off a bed and sustained a bump to the head. The call handler probes for more information about how the baby fell and who was looking after it at the time. She is told that the baby rolled off the bed. The call handler uses good listening skills and critical thinking to arrive at the conclusion that there may be a safeguarding issue. She realises that developmentally a six-week-old baby cannot roll over. She also concludes that even if the baby had accidentally rolled off, she should have been supervised. A safeguarding referral is made following a discussion about this with the caller. The child is also referred to the emergency department.

The child is seen in the emergency department but the father gives a different story about how the injury occurred. The father says that one of the younger children accidentally bumped the baby on the head with a toy. Staff within the emergency department accepted this as a plausible reason. However, as a result of the referral, a health visitor visits the family some days later. It is discovered that the baby's mother is suffering from severe depression and that the father is looking after the family's four children single-handedly. Appropriate family support is arranged as well as an urgent mental health assessment for the mother.

Scenario 2

Your organisation receives a call from a very distressed woman who states she is depressed and cannot go on any longer. She struggles to give you her location as she left home three hours earlier and has been walking around the town. Using your call handling skills you are able to establish a rapport with this caller; she finally informs you that she is on a small trading estate on the edge of town and is heading towards the railway track to end it all. She goes on to tell you that she cannot cope as she has three young children at home, all below school age. She has struggled to bring them up alone since her husband walked out eight months ago and she has no family or friends to support her. The previous morning she had received a letter from the local council stating that they would be starting eviction proceedings against her for non-payment of rent and that had been 'the final straw'. Your assessment results in an ambulance being dispatched.

> ### Time out activity – consider the following questions in relation to Scenario 2 before reading on
>
> - What safeguarding concerns does this call raise for you?
> - Given that an ambulance crew is being sent, is there any other action you would need to take regarding this call?

As well as the concerns for the welfare of the caller in Scenario 2, the welfare of her children must also be taken into consideration. This caller has indicated that three very young children have been left alone with no indication that they have any form of adult supervision.

Any safeguarding concerns heard by call handlers should always be reported, even if an ambulance is being dispatched or as in the case of the first scenario, the person has been referred to another professional. Callers who make contact in such a distressed state may act in a very unpredictable manner. The caller may suddenly end the call or their mobile phone battery could run out. She may move from the location she initially gave during the call or she may even make it to the railway tracks and succeed in her suicide attempt before the ambulance crew is able to locate her. The caller may also omit to inform the crew or hospital staff that her children are at home alone. Failure by a call handler to report the fact that three young children are in an extremely vulnerable position could cause a delay in them receiving the urgent assistance they require.

If any safeguarding issues are identified and an ambulance crew is attending, they should be made aware of any concerns, so that they can review these and take them into account.

Scenario 3

Sophie is 23. Along with her husband and three-month-old baby she has moved to a new part of the country. Sophie has no friends locally and her husband works long hours. She is struggling to cope with her young baby. In her haste to prepare supper for that evening's meal, she moves a pan of boiling water from the hob to the sink so she can drain some peas. She stumbles and splashes some boiling water over her baby who is in a baby bouncer on the floor.

Sophie dials 999 as her baby is screaming in pain. The call handler assesses the baby and provides information about what to do next.

Time out activity – consider the following question in relation to Scenario 3 before reading on
If you were the call handler involved, would you complete a safeguarding referral?

The call handler did not feel that a safeguarding referral was required because the injury was clearly the result of an unfortunate accident. There was no suspicion of any abuse or neglect. The call handler also worried that highlighting the call as a potential safeguarding issue might make life more difficult for Sophie.

Within days of Sophie's call, the call handler attended a safeguarding refresher workshop. He reflected on the call and felt he possibly should have reported this issue. He discussed it with the safeguarding lead and the call was referred using the organisation's procedure.

In the meantime, social services had already been alerted by the emergency department that treated the baby. Support had been arranged for Sophie and her health visitor had given her information about a local Young Mum's Network. Rather than making life more difficult for Sophie, the safeguarding referral meant appropriate support was put in place for the family. Fortunately, the emergency department acted appropriately and did report their concerns, however it must never be assumed that another agency will do this. You have no guarantee that the person will actually follow your advice and access the care you advised, just as there is no certainty that the receiving agency will be given the same information or indeed will pick up on any safeguarding issues. Everyone involved in a patient's care has a responsibility to report any concerns they pick up.

The referral to social services resulted in supportive measures being put in place with the potential to benefit Sophie and her child. This is the purpose of child safeguarding: to protect children and ensure they receive care which allows them to be safe and to flourish.

Scenario 4

A man calls your service reporting that he is the carer for his 85-year-old grandfather who has sustained facial injuries. The injuries are reported to be a 'gash just above the eye that won't stop bleeding'. You ask some questions to try and establish exactly what happened. The man gives what seem like quite vague answers such as 'He just tripped, it's no big deal, he's always doing it.' The caller seems to be slurring his words and you wonder if he may be under the influence of alcohol or drugs.

You ask to speak to the grandfather at which point the caller becomes annoyed and asks 'Why can't you just stop ******* prying and get an appointment for stitching sorted?' You manage to calm the caller down and he eventually puts his grandfather on the phone.

The patient is very quiet and withdrawn when he comes to the phone and keeps saying that he is fine. He keeps repeating it was just an accident; 'I fell over, I'm old and clumsy love, it was nobody's fault.' The grandson can be heard continuing to shout and swear in the background.

Time out activity – identifying concerns regarding a vulnerable adult
Take some time to think through the following questions before reading on:
• Is the grandfather a vulnerable adult?
• What issues would make you concerned that this is potentially an abusive situation?

The patient, who is very elderly, is being cared for by a grandson who presents as being aggressive and possibly under the influence of alcohol or drugs. These factors may make him susceptible to abuse.

Other issues that should give cause for concern include:

• The patient's demeanour which seems quiet and withdrawn.

• The caller and the patient seem to be minimising the injury.

• The caller is vague in his response rather than being clear about exactly what happened. If he had witnessed the injury he should be able to describe it. If he had not witnessed it, it would be entirely appropriate to say he did not know exactly what happened. Instead, he becomes angry when you try to establish more detail.

- The caller is reluctant to let you talk to his grandfather.
- The grandfather uses the phrase 'it was nobody's fault' even though the issue of blame had not been raised.
- The presence of an injury. This may, of course, have been entirely accidental, but on the other hand, it may have been the result of physical abuse. On the basis of the picture presented by the caller and patient, it would definitely not be correct to rule out the possibility of abuse.

Summary

Where safeguarding is concerned, the most important part of your role as a call handler is to listen, probe and act on any information that may suggest a vulnerable adult or child is at risk of, or being, abused.

Safeguarding can be a highly emotive topic for all concerned. This should be at the front of your mind when managing a situation where safeguarding is a concern. Try to remain calm, impartial and factual and keep the immediate safety of patients as your primary goal.

It is vital to be aware of the signs of abuse and to immediately raise any concerns you have through your local policy. Some of the tragic deaths of children and vulnerable adults who have died at the hands of serial abusers may not have occurred if professionals had acted on their concerns.

Be mindful that dealing with calls relating to potential safeguarding can be stressful. Make sure you get appropriate support and are able to talk such calls through with an appropriate person within your organisation.

Remember, if you are ever in any doubt as to whether a safeguarding referral would be appropriate, seek advice.

References and Further Reading

Material in this chapter has been reproduced from: Richard Pilbery and Kris Lethbridge, *Ambulance Care Practice*, Bridgwater: Class Publishing (2016), with kind permission from the authors.

CQC (2015), *Statement on CQC's roles and responsibilities for safeguarding children and adults*. Available at: https://www.cqc.org.uk/sites/default/files/20150710_CQC_New_Safeguarding_Statement.pdf (Accessed 20 June 2018).

Department for Education (2015). *Working together to safeguard children*. Available at: https://www.gov.uk/government/publications/working-together-to-safeguard-children--2 (Accessed 7 June 2018).

Department of Health (2016). *Multi-agency statutory guidance on female genital mutilation*. Available at: https://assets.publishing.service.gov.uk/government/uploads/system/uploads/attachment_data/file/512906/Multi_Agency_Statutory_Guidance_on_FGM__-_FINAL.pdf (Accessed 20 June 2018).

Department of Health (2011). *Safeguarding adults: the role of health services*. Available at: https://www.gov.uk/government/publications/safeguarding-adults-the-role-of-health-services (Accessed 7 June 2018).

Department of Health (2000). *No secrets: guidance on protecting vulnerable adults in care*. Available at: https://www.gov.uk/government/publications/no-secrets-guidance-on-protecting-vulnerable-adults-in-care (Accessed 7 June 2018).

Gov.UK (2008). *LSCB Haringey Serious Case Review: Baby Peter Connelly*. Available at: https://www.gov.uk/government/publications/haringey-local-safeguarding-children-board-first-serious-case-review-child-a (last accessed 9 April 2018).

Gov.UK (2015). *Working Together to Safeguard Children*. Available at: https://www.gov.uk/government/publications/working-together-to-safeguard-children--2 (last accessed 9 April 2018).

Calderdale Council (2016). *Safeguarding Adults*. Available at: www.calderdale.gov.uk/socialcare/safeguarding adults/index.html (last accessed 7 June 2018).

Home Affairs Committee (2012). *Introduction: Roots of Violent Radicalisation*. Available at: https://publications.parliament.uk/pa/cm201012/cmselect/cmhaff/1446/144603.htm (last accessed 9 April 2018).

May, T. (2011). *Prevent Strategy*. Norwich: TSO. Available at: www.gov.uk/government/uploads/system/uploads/attachment_data/file/97976/prevent-strategy-review.pdf (last accessed 8 December 2016).

NICE (2009). National Institute for Health and Care Excellence, 2009. *When to suspect child maltreatment*. Available at: http:// www.nice.org.uk/guidance/cg89 (Accessed 21 January 2015).

NHS Choices (2015). *Abuse and Neglect of Vulnerable Adults*. Available at: www.nhs.uk/Conditions/social-care-and-support-guide/Pages/vulnerable-people-abuse-safeguarding.aspx (last accessed 1 December 2016).

NHS (2018). *Safeguarding Adults*. Available at: www.myguideapps.com/nhs_safeguarding/default/safeguarding_adults/?nocache=0.000018013462501131894 (last accessed 1 December 2016).

NSPCC (2012). *Core Info: Bruises on Children*. Available at: www.nspcc.org.uk/globalassets/documents/advice-and-info/core-info-bruises-children.pdf (last accessed 21 April 2017).

NSPCC (2017a). *Safeguarding Children*. Available at: www.nspcc.org.uk/preventing-abuse/safeguarding/ (last accessed 1 December 2016).

NSPCC (2017b). *Signs, Symptoms and Effects for Different Types of Abuse* [Online]. Available at: www.nspcc.org.uk/preventing-abuse/signs-symptoms-effects/ (last accessed 21 April 2017).

Pilbery, R. and Lethbridge, K. (2016). *Ambulance Care Practice*. Bridgwater: Class Publishing.

Safeguarding Matters (2011). *Abuse of Vulnerable Adults*. [Online]. Available at: www.safeguardingmatters.co.uk/the-new-disclosure-and-vetting-service/in-the-news/recent-cases-relating-to-vulnerable-adults/ (last accessed 1 December 2016).

Telegraph (2009). *Lord Laming's review of Baby P failures*. Available at: www.telegraph.co.uk/news/uknews/baby-p/5283897/Lord-Lamings-review-of-Baby-P-failures.html (last accessed 1 December 2016).

The National Archives (2014). *The Care Act 2014*. Available at: http://www.legislation.gov.uk/ukpga/2014/23/contents/enacted (last accessed 9 April 2018).

The NHS Safeguarding App is a resource for healthcare professionals to increase their awareness and understanding of safeguarding requirements. This is available for IOS and Android devices. Available at: https://play.google.com/store/apps/details?id=com.antbits.nhsSafeguardingGuide&hl=en_GB (last accessed 9 April 2018).

Chapter 7: **Mental Health and Telephone Triage**

Learning Objectives

By the end of this chapter you will be able to:

- Define what is meant by 'mental health'
- Explain a range of common mental health disorders
- Explain a range of severe mental health disorders
- Summarise a range of other mental health-related conditions such as dementia and self-harm
- State appropriate sources of help and support for people suffering from mental health issues
- Describe a range of call handling skills for helping people with mental health issues
- Explain how to manage calls relating to suicide
- List a range of myths and facts related to suicide.

Introduction

Mental health is a very complex area, but it can affect anyone from all walks of life. One of the key messages here is not to be frightened of it. There are many factors that can contribute to becoming mentally ill: head trauma, a life-threatening or chronic physical illness, abusing drugs and alcohol, social deprivation, life events, etc. Our brains can either function in a way that allows us to take part in the normal aspects of daily life – going to work, learning, playing sports, socialising with family or friends – or it can be affected by conditions that prevent us from living a full and happy existence.

The aim of this chapter is to give you a baseline understanding of the major mental health conditions you may encounter in your role. It is not intended to make you an expert, but rather to raise your awareness and understanding with the aim of helping you deal sensitively with the calls you will undoubtedly receive.

What is Mental Health?

The World Health Organization describes Mental Health as:

'A state of well-being in which every individual realises his or her own potential, can cope with the normal stresses of life, can work productively and fruitfully, and is able to make a contribution to her or his community.'
(Source: World Health Organization, July 2015)

It might be helpful to consider that we can be physically healthy but sometimes suffer from an illness or condition that affects our body. The same can apply to our brain, and it's surprisingly common.

Some physical conditions, for instance a cold, are time limited. We may feel rotten, with a runny nose, sore throat and possibly a headache, but with good self-care, such as taking over-the-counter pain relief, drinking plenty of fluids, and getting rest, the cold will clear up by itself. However, sometimes the condition we are suffering from needs treatment from a healthcare professional for us to recover. Very occasionally, despite medical intervention, we have to learn to live with a less than perfectly functioning body.

The same applies to mental illness. In 2014, one in three adults with conditions such as anxiety and depression surveyed in England were accessing mental health treatment [Adult Psychiatric Morbidity Survey, 2014]. Despite the increasing numbers and the fact that depression is one of the best documented and well researched mental health illnesses, it's a subject that is often not talked about; sadly there is still a lot of stigma and taboo surrounding the condition.

Common Mental Health Disorders

Depression

Depression lowers your mood and can make you feel hopeless, worthless, unmotivated and exhausted. It can affect self-esteem, sleep, appetite and libido. Depression can also interfere with daily activities and, sometimes, a person's physical health. In its mildest form, depression can mean just being in low spirits. It doesn't stop you leading a normal life, but makes everything harder to do and seem less worthwhile. At its most severe, major depression (clinical depression) can be life-threatening, and make you feel suicidal.

Post-Natal Depression (PND)

This is a form of deep and longer-term depression that some women experience after giving birth. It affects around 10–15% of new mothers. It usually develops within six weeks of giving birth, can come on gradually or suddenly and can range from mild to very severe. Women with post-natal depression may experience one or more of the following symptoms:

- Feeling sad, low and tearful for no apparent reason.
- Feeling worthless or hopeless about the future.
- Tiredness.
- Inability to cope.
- Irritability, anger and guilt.
- Hostility/indifference to their partner and/or the baby.
- Poor concentration.
- Sleep problems.
- Reduced appetite.
- Lack of interest in sex.
- Thoughts about death.

Anxiety

Anxiety is the main symptom of several conditions, including panic disorder and post-traumatic stress disorder. There are several types of anxiety and panic disorders.

Generalised Anxiety Disorder (GAD)

This is a condition diagnosed when the patient has felt anxious and fearful for a long time, without there being any particular focus for the anxiety.

Obsessive Compulsive Disorder (OCD)

This is characterised by obsessive thoughts, which compel a person to behave in certain ways. For example, a person with OCD may have obsessive thoughts about hygiene, compelling them to wash their hands repeatedly.

Post-traumatic Stress disorder (PTSD)

This can arise following highly traumatic events such as war, serious accident, rape or violence. PTSD causes flashbacks and dreams recalling the event and can trigger the same feelings as were originally experienced.

Panic Disorder

Everybody experiences feelings of anxiety and panic at certain times during their life. It is a perfectly natural response, particularly when you are in a threatening situation. However, for people with panic disorder, intense feelings of anxiety and panic occur regularly and sometimes randomly. A panic attack occurs when the body experiences a rush of intense psychological and physical symptoms such as extreme fear and apprehension, accompanied by nausea, trembling and palpitations.

Severe Mental Health Conditions

Bipolar Disorder

This condition is characterised by severe mood swings. These phases usually last several weeks or months and are far beyond what most of us experience. The phases are:

- *Low* or '*depressive*': feelings of intense depression and despair.
- *High* or '*manic*': feelings of intense wellbeing, energy and optimism which can be so extreme that it causes the patient to make impulsive and often unwise decisions. During this phase, it is not uncommon for people to believe strange things about themselves and behave in embarrassing, harmful and occasionally dangerous ways.
- *Mixed*: depressed mood with feelings of agitation/restlessness.

Psychosis

This is where a person loses touch with reality. They may feel paranoid, hallucinate, hear voices and have delusions or confused thoughts. Psychosis can occur with bipolar disorder and is a major part of the condition commonly known as schizophrenia. People can also experience psychotic episodes due to severe stress or depression or as a result of drug or alcohol use.

It is believed that there is a particular link to cannabis. People who have a history of mental illness in their family are more at risk from a psychotic episode.

Someone going through psychosis is said to be experiencing a 'psychotic episode'. Often the first episode occurs in their early teens or twenties. They may have one episode or continue to have them throughout their lives. People with psychosis may experience distressing symptoms such as:

- Hallucinations – hearing voices no-one else hears, seeing things that aren't there, or feeling, smelling or tasting unusual sensations with no obvious cause.
- Believing others can influence their thoughts, or they can influence the thoughts of others or control events.
- Believing they are being watched, followed or persecuted by others or that their life is in danger.
- Feeling their thoughts have sped up or slowed down.
- Thinking or talking in a confused way.
- Withdrawal from normal everyday life and activities and a flat, apathetic demeanor.

Other Mental Health-related Conditions

Dementia

This is a syndrome (a group of related symptoms) associated with an ongoing decline of the brain and its abilities. Alzheimer's disease is a form of dementia.

Symptoms include:

- Memory loss, especially problems with memory for recent events, such as forgetting messages, remembering routes or names, and asking questions repetitively.
- Problems with thinking speed and mental agility.
- Increasing difficulties with tasks and activities that require organisation and planning.
- Becoming confused in unfamiliar environments.
- Difficulty finding the right words.
- Difficulty with numbers and/or handling money in shops.
- Changes in personality and mood, including depression.

Self-harm

This is an umbrella term that covers a wide range of behaviours, the end result being that the behaviour intentionally causes harm. It is often understood to be a physical response to emotional pain and is a very complex area. The behaviour can also be be highly addictive.

Self-harming behaviour is not the same as suicidal behaviour, and this is a distinction you will be required to make, with the support of the system you are using. Although there are links between self-harm and suicide, people who self-harm are generally not trying to end their life, but rather to cope with the stresses and strains they are facing.

Self-harm results in about 150,000 attendances at emergency departments each year. It is one of the top five causes of acute medical admission. Rates of self-harm in the UK have increased over the past decade and are among the highest in Europe. It is thought that around 13% of young people may try to hurt themselves on purpose at some point between the ages of 11 and 16, but the actual figure could be much higher [NICE, 2014].

Any injury or harm to the body that is caused deliberately would be considered self-harming, such as:

- Cutting, burning or scratching skin
- Punching, or hitting
- Poisoning with tablets or toxic chemicals
- Abusing alcohol or drugs
- Deliberately starving or binge eating
- Excessively exercising
- Asphyxiation
- Hair pulling.

Alcohol and Substance Misuse

Using alcohol to excess or taking illegal drugs is often closely linked with several mental health conditions. Some people use this behaviour to cope with an existing illness, but their use can make the condition worse (e.g. there is a link between smoking marijuana and psychotic episodes).

Abusing alcohol can have disastrous effects on our physical and mental health. It may be a coping strategy to a life event (such as a relationship break up) but can quickly spiral out of control, leading to severe conditions.

Getting Help for Mental Health Conditions

One of the most difficult issues when someone has a mental health condition is taking the first step to get help. It can be very hard to admit to yourself that you have a problem and to seek help. People who have a loved one who is suffering are often the first to spot something isn't quite right, but sometimes feel powerless to provide support or really aren't sure where to go for help.

A good first step for someone suffering from problems with their mental health is to speak to a GP. They may be able to diagnose the condition/illness and, having done that, advise and provide guidance as to the most appropriate treatment.

General Practitioners

GPs are the gateway to referring patients on to secondary mental health services, (e.g. access to a psychiatrist, or psychologist, local community services, etc). If required, they can also provide treatment in the way of drug therapies (antidepressants, beta blockers for anxiety, etc.) and talking therapies. Some GP practices have a counsellor working within the service. For some people, talking through their issues can be hugely helpful.

Mental Health Crisis Teams

These are found around the country (although not in all areas) and are staffed by experienced healthcare professionals. Often the team will comprise doctors, specialist nurses and therapists, who provide a holistic approach. Some services allow patients to self-refer. Potential patients reaching out for help may be invited to attend a telephone interview with a trained counsellor, who will talk through the issues and advise of the range of services available in the area.

Charities and Voluntary Organisations

There are a wide range of charitable and voluntary agencies which can provide help to people struggling with issues associated with mental health. These include national organisations such as Mind, the Samaritans and Sane Line. There will also be smaller organisations specialising in mental health in local areas. For some people, accessing these types of organisations, which are often run by well trained and supported volunteers, can provide a life line when NHS services are not available. Some telephone support services are available 24/7. The NHS is recognising the added benefit that this sort of support can provide on the road to regaining better health, and is working collaboratively with them to provide a safety network for vulnerable/unwell people.

Call Handling Skills for Helping People with Mental Health Issues

It can be distressing talking to people who are experiencing mental health problems, particularly if they display strong emotions such as anxiety, sadness, hopelessness or anger. Thinking this through beforehand is really helpful. A key principle to bear in mind is that it is vital that the caller understands you have 'heard the message'. Every call is different but there are some key techniques that can be used to help you manage emotion over the telephone.

Five key techniques for managing strong emotion over the telephone

1. Empathise

   When we are experiencing strong emotions, it can help to know that someone understands how we're feeling. This is often enough to help a person regain some emotional equilibrium. Empathy statements are ways of showing a caller that you have recognised the way they feel. Whilst the list is not intended to be exhaustive, the following phrases may be useful. 'That must be very difficult for you' or 'It sounds as if you are having a tough time' or 'That must be very upsetting for you'.

2. Use your voice skilfully

   Your voice is one of your strongest assets within telephone triage and you can use it to demonstrate care, concern and warmth. Use your voice to create a 'safe space' for the caller or patient to tell you how they are feeling.

3. Acknowledge the caller's need

   Let the person know that you've heard the reason for their call by summarising what you think they are saying. When someone is in distress it can be a powerful thing to be truly heard and listened to. Use reflective or summarising statements to reflect back to the caller what you have heard, for example 'So you have been feeling very low for a couple of days' or 'I heard you say that life isn't worth living…'. This technique also gives the person a chance to address any misunderstandings.

4. Use the blameless apology

    Blameless apologies do not place blame on anyone or anything. They are a professional way of apologising for something that has upset the caller without actually agreeing with them and making excuses. Examples include:

    'I'm sorry that happened' or 'I'm sorry you feel that way'.

    This is a technique used within a customer service context, but it can be very useful in helping to disarm any strong emotion over the telephone.

5. Use positive factual statements

    These allow you to offer callers professional reassurance without making unrealistic promises. It can help to combine these with empathetic statements to make it clear that you understand their situation. For example:

    'It sounds like you are having a very difficult time at the moment. I can hear how upset you are. What I am going to do is ask you some questions about how things are right now, so that I can help you with the next steps.'

Managing Calls Relating to Suicide

It is likely that, within your role as a call handler, you will manage calls associated with suicide. This may be because someone has attempted suicide or because they are contemplating taking their own life.

According to the Samaritans, there were over 4,500 suicides in England in 2012. However, the true number is probably underestimated. The age groups most at risk of suicide are 40–44 in males and 50–54 in females.

You may hear people expressing the view that if a person is serious about killing themselves, there is nothing that you can do to prevent it over the telephone. However, this is not the case. Feeling suicidal is often a temporary state of mind. Although someone may feel down or distressed

for a sustained period, the actual suicidal crisis can be relatively short term. If a person receives appropriate support and treatment, they may recover.

Your role in helping them access appropriate care and support is crucial, so never underestimate the vital role you have to play in the management of people expressing a desire to end their life. It is also important to understand that the majority of people who feel suicidal do not actually want to die, but they do want to be free of their emotional pain and suffering.

There can be many reasons why a person may feel suicidal. It could be that they are living with a range of mental health conditions such as depression and anxiety. They might have been through a significant life event, a relationship break up, the death of a loved one, been diagnosed with a serious illness, drinking heavily or using recreational drugs, worried about exam results, suffering physical/sexual/emotional abuse, feeling lonely, or struggling with their sexuality. There may be a family history of suicide.

Myths and facts about suicide

The following section is taken from the Samaritans website and provides an insight into many of the myths surrounding suicide.

Myth: *You have to be mentally ill to even think about suicide.*

Fact: From time to time, many people have thoughts about ending their life. It may be a fleeting 'it would be so much easier if I wasn't here' which comes into their head and then disappears, or a thought that is with them on a regular basis. Not all people who die by suicide have a diagnosed mental health condition, although some do and their condition is often serious.

Myth: *People who talk about suicide aren't serious and won't go through with it. It is just a 'cry for help'.*

Fact: People who choose to end their life have often told someone, possibly a relative or a close friend that they do not want to carry on living. They may have posted about how they feel on social media sites. It has been recorded in coroners' reports that of those who are successful in killing themselves, some visited their GP in the four weeks leading up to their death. It is a common misconception that if someone says 'I just want to die', they are attention seeking. Consider for a moment what they are saying. If you hear that phrase, it's vital to listen seriously to anyone who is talking about suicide.

Myth: *Talking about suicide is a bad idea, as it might give someone the idea to try it.*

Fact: Sadly suicide is still considered as a taboo by society. So people feel they can't talk to their family or friends about how they are feeling and don't want to upset them or consider themselves to be a burden, so they don't share how they are feeling.

Myth: *People who are suicidal want to die.*

Fact: The majority of people who feel suicidal do not actually want to die. The way they are feeling may be short-lived. They may have reached a crisis point, for example someone who is bereaved may feel like this on the anniversary of their loved one's death. In the early stages of a relationship break up or the diagnosis of a terminal condition, they do not want the life they have. The distinction may seem small, but it is in fact very important. Talking about other options is a key factor in helping.

Myth: *Men should display a 'stiff upper lip' and just get on with it.*

Fact: Suicide is the most common cause of death for men under the age of 35, and the group that is most at risk is between 45 and 49. Many men have been brought up to believe that it's not manly or is a sign of weakness to display emotion or ask for help.

(Source: The Samaritans)

Time out activity – call handling skills for managing suicidal callers

We first met Hugo in Chapter Two. Here he gives us his perspective about what happened on the day he attempted suicide.

'I was feeling so low that day. It felt like my life was crumbling around me and that everyone would be better off without me. Losing my job was the last straw. It was like a physical pain and I just wanted the pain to end. I don't really remember much about cutting my wrist, but I do remember the look on Sally's face. She called 999 and I felt so angry.

The woman I spoke to tried to be friendly and reassuring but I was a total mess. I feel terrible about the way I spoke to her. When I was raging and shouting, she kept repeating my name quite quietly … 'Hugo, I'm here to help you. Hugo, let me help'.

She picked up that I was in a terrible state and she gave me the time and space to rant and then to tell her a little of how I was feeling. I can't remember much about what she said, but I can remember she was calm and somehow it sounded like she cared.

Her voice sounded soothing and warm. That made a difference for some reason – that a stranger didn't judge me and that I mattered enough for her listen. When I explained the desperate mess my life was in, I think she said something like 'That sounds really awful Hugo'. I felt, I dunno, I suppose validated in some way.

She really did seem to listen and it was this that persuaded me to let the ambulance come. I don't know if she'd have sent it anyway, but it was probably the right thing to do. Things are still hard, but I am starting to see that it might not always be so bleak, and here I am, still fighting.'

Before reading on, take a few minutes to think about the skills the call handler used to manage Hugo's call

How you manage a call related to suicide will vary greatly depending on the circumstances of the caller so it is not possible to offer a one-size-fits-all process. However, there are some general techniques and approaches that might help.

Techniques and approaches for dealing with patients expressing suicidal thoughts

Try to avoid:

- Any tendency to criticise or make assumptions about the person's situation.
- Prejudging or not taking seriously the patient's commitment to suicide.
- Negative or demeaning language. In particular, avoid the term 'commit' suicide. The phrase developed when suicide was considered to be both a criminal act and a sin. It is fine to say suicide, just avoid the 'commit' part.
- Asking 'why' questions. Too many 'why' questions can feel like an interrogation, especially if the person is not easily able to articulate why they feel like they do.
- Sounding patronising or insincere. Phrases such as 'I don't want you to do anything silly' can come across as glib.
- Giving the impression you are not interested or 'have heard it all before'.
- Making unrealistic promises or agreeing to demands. For example, it would be inappropriate to make promises about being seen in the emergency department by a specialist mental health practitioner, because this might not actually be possible.
- Quickly offering solutions.

What may help?

- Keep safety uppermost in your mind – this includes the patient, any bystanders and any professionals sent to the scene.
- Take threats very seriously.
- Think carefully about how you come across. It can help to think about how you would like a dearly loved relative or friend to be treated in this situation. You should strive to demonstrate understanding and uncritical acceptance, along with respect and empathy. Make sure you demonstrate that you care and are listening.
- Use clear, unambiguous language and do not be afraid of asking direct questions about their intentions, such as whether they have made a plan and whether they have the means to carry this out. Do not be afraid of words and phrases like 'ending your life' and 'killing yourself'.
- Talk slowly and clearly and check understanding. Allow the patient to have their turn talking.
- Personalise the call – actively listen to the details of what is said and use them. Use the patient's name.
- Use the caller's language by reflecting and summarising what they have said.
- Allow silences.
- Allow the caller to vent their emotions and remember that any anger or other strong emotion is not really directed at you – it's a product of the person's suffering.
- Recognise that calls relating to suicide can be very stressful. Make sure you get appropriate support during the call if required, as well as afterwards.

The Mental Health Act 1983

The Mental Health Act 1983 is the law which sets out when a person can be admitted, detained and treated in hospital against their wishes for reasons relating to their mental health. This is also known as being 'sectioned', because there are different sections to the act which apply in different circumstances.

People are only sectioned when they are putting their own safety, or someone else's safety, at risk. Some sections of the Mental Health Act mean that treatment without consent can be given.

Sometimes you may receive calls from healthcare professionals or the police requesting that an ambulance be dispatched for someone who needs admitting, detaining or treating under the Mental Health Act. Understanding some of the relevant sections of the Act, which are outlined briefly below, can give you more confidence in dealing with these professionals, however it is not your role in these circumstances to question whether the ambulance is required.

Section 2 allows a person to be admitted to hospital for an assessment of their mental health and receive any necessary treatment for up to 28 days. An admission to hospital under section 2 is usually used when the person has not been assessed in hospital before or when their last assessment was a considerable time ago.

Section 3 allows a person to be detained in hospital for treatment. Detention under section 3 is indicated where the person is well known to mental health services, or following admission under section 2. Treatment might be necessary for their health, their safety or for the protection of other people.

Section 4 is used in emergency situations, where a person is detained in hospital for an assessment of their mental health for a shorter period of time. Unlike a section 2, which needs two medical recommendations, it only needs the recommendation of one doctor. It is used when carrying out a section 2 assessment would create an undesirable delay which may be detrimental to the health/safety of the patient or other people.

Section 5 allows a doctor or nurse to stop you from leaving hospital. It can also be used if you are having treatment in a general hospital for a physical condition.

Section 135 is used to take a person to a place of safety for a mental health assessment. This is used when the patient is in a private place and they are not able to care for themselves or are not being taken care of properly. This section allows the police to enter a person's home.

Section 136 is used to take a person to a place of safety when they are in a public place. They can do this if they think the person has a mental illness and are in need of care. A place of safety can be a hospital or a police station.

Summary

Remember, these calls can be really challenging. Make sure you recognise the impact they may have and be proactive in getting the appropriate support. In order to be able to do your job effectively, to remain focused and give every caller/patient the best service on every call, it is vital that you look after yourself.

It is important to know what sources of support you have within your organisation. During your shift, if you need time out to debrief after a difficult call, do you know who to talk to? Do you know the policy for taking time off the phone if you are not due for a break? Getting support with a difficult call might involve seeking guidance from a senior colleague during the call or debriefing with someone afterwards. You may need to take some time out before moving on to the next call – maybe this is where a few minutes of mindful breathing could be useful. This technique is explained in Chapter Ten. You might also want to listen to the call afterwards to reflect on how you managed it, if this facility is available to you. Post-traumatic stress disorder is a condition which is all too common among emergency staff, including those in 999 and 111 call centres. It is important that you seek early help if you ever feel affected by a call that you have been involved with.

Whatever you choose to do, make sure you prioritise your own wellbeing so as to avoid becoming 'burned out', or taking any unresolved issues into the next call. It is also important to be very mindful of the need for confidentiality: make sure you deal with things before you leave work, as you should not be talking about cases with anyone outside of work.

References and Further Reading

Adult Psychiatric Morbidity Survey (2014). *Survey of Mental Health and Wellbeing, England.* Available at: http://digital.nhs.uk/catalogue/PUB21748 (last accessed 10 April 2018).

NICE (2014). *Using NICE CG16 Self-harm Guidance to Improve Psychosocial Assessment of Patients Following Self Harm.* Available at: https://www.nice.org.uk/sharedlearning/using-nice-cg16-self-harm-guidance-to-improve-psychosocial-assessment-of-patients-following-self-harm (last accessed 9 April 2018).

The Samaritans (2014). Available at: www.samaritans.org/how-we-can-help-you/myths-about-suicide (last accessed 10 April 2018).

Chapter 8: Special Considerations

Learning Objectives

By the end of this chapter you will be able to:

- Describe the challenges presented when triaging different caller groups, including children, elderly callers, frequent callers, patients receiving end of life care and callers with little or no English
- Discuss safe and appropriate strategies for dealing with different patient groups
- Define the terms 'learning disability' and 'autism'
- Describe the causes of learning disability and autism
- Explain the needs of a person with a learning disability or autism in the context of telephone triage
- Describe how learning disabilities and autism lead to inequality in healthcare
- Describe how you may need to adapt your methods of communication when assisting people with learning disabilities and autism
- Describe how learning disabilities and autism influence a person's vulnerability.

Introduction

One of the challenges of telephone triage is that you will have no idea what the call will be about when you answer the phone. This can be exciting and prevent the role from becoming monotonous, but the flip side is that it can be stressful because it is not possible to predict the type of call, or prepare for a difficult or upsetting situation.

This means that from the start of your shift and right up until your last call, you need to pay full attention. There are some groups of patients or callers who may require you to adapt your approach slightly: in this chapter we are going to examine some of the challenges you might encounter, and possible solutions.

Children

Children's bodies are different to those of adults and change throughout childhood. For example, children's immune responses aren't fully developed making them prone to minor infections. Young children may deteriorate quite quickly when poorly and their developing organs can also be more prone to long-term damage than those of adults. This means that children sometimes need more urgent treatment than adults with similar symptoms.

Children also suffer from a different range of conditions to those commonly seen in adults. Heart disease is less common in children, since most heart disease occurs over time as a result of the ageing process. This means that in assessing something like chest pain, different questions need to be asked of children and adults.

A child's symptoms are often described by another person. This information may be detailed and accurate or vague and unreliable. An adult can usually differentiate between earache, a sore throat or a neck pain but with young children who are pre-verbal, it can be difficult to get a clear picture of exactly what the symptoms are, as there may be considerable overlap.

Speaking to a child may be a familiar occurrence if you have children or younger siblings, however, for some call handlers, this is new territory. There are no fixed guidelines regarding the age of a child that you can ask to speak to. Some children will relish the chance to tell you about their symptoms, and you will gain valuable information from talking to them.

Others may be shy and not want to talk to a strange person on the phone, so it is very much a matter of judgement on your part. You can always take the lead from the carer calling on behalf of the child, by asking if it is possible to speak to them. Clearly it would not be appropriate to try to speak to a child who is very upset or feeling particularly unwell.

Keep your language simple and straightforward and don't speak down to a younger caller. Allow the child time to answer your questions and ensure that they understand. You may have to rephrase the way you ask them, and apply critical thinking. Am I certain that this child really understands what I am asking them, and do I understand their answers?'

Depending on the age of your caller, you may need to use 'lay' terms for body parts, for example, tummy rather than abdomen. It can be helpful to mirror what the child is saying, but a note of caution here: any notes you make during a triage are part of the patient record.

The child may say 'my tummy hurts when I do a poo', but it would be more appropriate to record 'abdominal pain when passing a bowel motion' in the call record. If you are going to quote something verbatim, you should use speech marks to indicate that this is exactly what the patient said.

A child might be shy talking about certain things such as their genital area and problems in that region, so you need to be extra sensitive in this case. A soft, warm, caring tone will often encourage a young person to tell you what is going on for them. Believe what they are saying and, if in doubt, check out what is happening carefully and whether there is an adult there who you can speak to.

When assessing children we must always be alert to the issues of abuse. Although any age group can be subject to abuse, children are more vulnerable than most adults [Department of Health, 2015]. Children under one are more vulnerable to abuse than any other age group [NSPCC, 2015]. All health service staff have a responsibility to safeguard and promote the welfare of children. Make sure you are really familiar with your child protection policy and procedures and know what to do when you come across a child who you think may be at risk.

Elderly Callers

Older patients are often very long suffering, and will only call for medical advice when things have become quite serious. You may find that they are quite apologetic, and a common phrase you might hear is 'sorry to bother you, I know there are people far worse off than me'.

The problem with this stoic approach is that often older patients don't contact a service until things have become quite serious, so be prepared to action their symptoms appropriately and in a timely manner.

There are several things to consider when speaking with older patients:

- how you greet them and what you call them during the call
- any hearing impairment
- dealing with confusion
- any visual impairment
- any mobility or dexterity impairment.

Many older people were brought up to only use a first name if invited to. It may be prudent to ask 'do you mind if I call you Imran, Mr Patel?' for example. If the caller tells you that they can't hear very well, consider how you are speaking to them. Slowing down your speech and making sure you pronounce your words clearly will help. You may need to spell words out. Ensure that the mouthpiece of your headset is correctly positioned.

If the patient is visually impaired they may not be able to answer questions regarding medication spelling, skin tone, or if their eyes have turned yellow, for example. They may have someone with them, who can support the patient to answer your questions.

Mobility or dexterity issues may mean that the patient can't move around as freely as an able bodied person, so be aware if you are asking them to do certain things, such as requesting that they put their chin on their chest.

If the patient is confused, consider what they are struggling with. They can usually tell you what is wrong, but may be uncertain about information such as times and dates. Being patient will help and you may need to think about phrasing things in a different way, or getting assistance.

Be mindful about whether an older person is vulnerable or possibly at risk of elder abuse from what the patient or carer is telling you. As with children, it is important to flag up any concerns, and to know your safeguarding polices regarding older people.

Frequent Callers

Everyone who contacts your service will have a need, and sometimes certain factors come into play which means that a caller will contact the service frequently. They may have complex medical needs, or have a mental health condition, such as anxiety.

Your voice may be the only one the patient has heard today, or for several days. Loneliness and isolation can exacerbate physical and mental ill health, and the patient may rely on your service for some form of human interaction.

One of the common pitfalls is to think 'oh it's … again. They always say they have back pain and want to speak to a clinician'. Whilst this may be true, the very nature of telephone triage means that we can only use the responses to the questions we ask the patient.

It isn't the role of a call handler to decide whether the patient is being honest in their responses, and if after some gentle probing they are insistent that they are in pain, you should proceed accordingly.

You must always refer to your local procedures for dealing with frequent callers, and where necessary, take advice from a clinical colleague. Remember that just like anyone else, frequent callers deserve to be treated in a professional, empathetic manner, regardless of how often they call.

Patients Receiving End of Life Care

Calls regarding patients who are terminally ill and receiving palliative care can be distressing. Although death is very much part of life, it is something that not everyone feels comfortable talking about. Those patients who are coming to the end of their journey may have very specific requirements.

They will often be under the care of specialist teams, with a detailed care plan, listing their medication requirements, chosen place of death and what to do when things deteriorate. For example, there may be extra pain relief medication in an injectable form stored in the fridge if the patient has chosen to die at home.

A key consideration here is empathy. The relative or carer may be quite emotional, so allow them the space to explain what they need. A simple empathetic statement such as 'I can hear you are very upset' shows the caller that you have acknowledged the emotion and they aren't talking to a robot. It is vital that you are familiar with your service's policies regarding this subject, because you may need to take advice or transfer the call appropriately.

Callers with Little or No English

The UK is ethnically diverse, and you will receive calls to your service from patients or carers where English is not their first language. In some cases, they won't be able to speak English at all, so you will need to use a translation service. You should have received training on how to do this, but if you are not certain, then consult your line manager.

Points to consider:

- Usually if the patient can't speak any English, they will be able to tell you what language they speak.
- Speak to the translator as if you are speaking to the patient, for example 'can you tell me where the pain is?' rather than 'can you ask her where the pain is?'
- Calls using a translator will take longer.

Remember that if you need to transfer the call to a clinical colleague, or end up calling an ambulance, inform the other parties that the patient does not speak English.

Learning Disabilities, Autism or Both

A learning disability is defined as a reduced intellectual ability and difficulty with everyday activities – for example household tasks, socialising or managing money – which affects someone for their whole life [Mencap, 2015]. Learning disability includes the presence of [DoH, 2001]:

- A significantly reduced ability to understand new or complex information, to learn new skills (impaired intelligence), with
- A reduced ability to cope independently (impaired social functioning),
- Which started before adulthood, with a lasting effect on development.

It is thought that up to 350,000 people in the UK have severe learning disabilities and this figure is increasing [NHS Choices, 2013].

The term autism will be used throughout this chapter as an umbrella term for all autistic spectrum conditions, including Asperger's syndrome. Autism is a life-long developmental disorder which affects how a person communicates with and relates to other people and how they experience the world around them.

It is thought that over 1.1% of the population have autism [The National Autistic Society, 2018].

It is important to remember that many people with learning disabilities, autism or both also have related hidden impairments such as attention deficit hyperactivity disorder (ADHD), dyspraxia, dyslexia and language impairments as well as associated mental health conditions. Learning disabilities are categorised as mild, moderate, severe or profound [Holland, 2011]. As with all conditions, the way in which any individual is challenged by their disability will be unique to them. Many people diagnosed with learning disabilities will be able to lead largely independent lives, whereas others may need more significant help and support.

Throughout the remainder of this section and for ease of discussion, we will refer to people with 'learning disabilities and autism'. However, the call handler should be aware that both may co-exist.

Causes of Learning Disabilities

There are four main causes that are responsible for learning disabilities [Holland, 2011]:

- Genetics
- Events before birth
- Events during birth
- Events after birth.

Genetics

Chromosomal conditions, such as Down's syndrome or Fragile X syndrome, are not in themselves learning disabilities, but they do frequently cause them.

Events Before Birth

Infections that a mother suffers during pregnancy can be transmitted to the fetus, leading to developmental problems and learning disabilities. Other maternal factors, including dietary deficiencies, excessive alcohol consumption during the pregnancy and endocrine disorders such as phenylketonuria can also cause learning disabilities.

Events During Birth

If during a traumatic or difficult delivery a baby's oxygen supply is interrupted for a significant period of time, brain damage may occur which can cause a learning disability.

Events After Birth

In the early years of life, a child is susceptible to many factors which may cause long-term impairment and learning disabilities. Examples of these include infections, particularly meningitis or encephalitis, and traumatic brain injuries, sustained by falls, road traffic accidents or non-accidental injuries.

Causes of Autism

There are various theories as to what causes autism. Most researchers believe that autism has a variety of causes, that it has a biological basis and a strong genetic component [Medical Research Council, 2001].

Autism is a spectrum condition. This means that people with autism will share certain difficulties in terms of their communication, how they relate to others and how they see the world, but they will be affected in different ways. Some people with autism say that the world feels overwhelming; this can cause them considerable anxiety.

Access to Healthcare

As a call handler you will undoubtedly come across people with learning disabilities and/or autism. You must always assess any patient with learning disabilities as an individual. It's important to remember that a learning disability does not necessarily make a person incapable of making decisions about their own care needs. Those with learning disabilities and autism have the same rights as everyone else. These rights are detailed within the Human Rights Act 1998. This obviously includes the right to access appropriate healthcare; however, this is not without its challenges for people with learning disabilities or autism.

People with learning disabilities and autism are more likely to have additional health problems. This includes a higher incidence of weight-related problems, mental health issues and respiratory diseases. People with learning disabilities and autism often have poorer health outcomes due to inequalities in healthcare. This means that they die younger and sometimes in situations where their death could have been prevented if they had received better-quality care [Mencap (2015) and Westminster Autism Commission (2016)].

In 2007, Mencap released the report *Death by Indifference*, which detailed institutional discrimination within the NHS against people with learning disabilities. The main findings of that report were that:

- The NHS viewed people with learning disabilities as a low priority.
- Many healthcare professionals did not understand much about learning disabilities.
- Families and carers of people with learning disabilities were frequently not properly consulted and involved.
- Health professionals often had a poor understanding of capacity and consent, particularly how this should be applied to those with learning disabilities.
- Health professionals relied inappropriately on their estimates of a person's quality of life.
- The complaints system within the NHS was often ineffectual, time-consuming and inaccessible.

Due to increasing awareness about these issues, over 200 hospitals have now signed up to the 'Getting it Right' charter; a set of principles for providing patients with learning disabilities with the best care possible.

Working within telephone triage, you will inevitably encounter people with learning disabilities and autism. Sometimes these conditions may be disclosed and at other times not. As with any caller, your role is to try and empower them to receive the healthcare they need. If you become aware or suspect that someone has autism or a learning disability which may prove a barrier to them getting the help they need, make sure you do not end the call without feeling confident that they are going to be able to access the care they need. Ask someone senior for some guidance if you are unsure about how to help or what to suggest. Sometimes relatively straightforward things can make a difference, such as making a GP appointment for them, rather than advising they do it themselves, or helping them plan their journey to their local GP surgery.

As a healthcare worker, you have a responsibility to make all reasonable adjustments necessary to ensure that patients with learning disabilities and autism receive the same standard of care as any other patients. Modifications will be unique based on the situation but, very importantly, you will need to adjust your communication techniques.

Every individual with learning disabilities and autism will have their own unique way of communicating. For patients with a mild learning disability, you may be able to communicate as you usually would, just ensuring that you use language that is not overly complex or difficult to understand. For patients with more severe or profound learning disabilities, it is likely you will need to conduct the call through a third party.

Tips for call management if a learning disability is declared or suspected

- If the person has difficulty communicating, consider that they might have a learning disability, autism and/or another condition.
- Ask the person if they have a Health or Hospital Passport. This can contain a lot of the information you need which the person may find hard to remember.
- If someone says they have a learning disability and/or autism, ask them how you can make the call easier for them.
- Try and ensure the interaction is free from distractions.
- Ask simple questions and do not rush the call. Give them time to answer.
- If the person is with someone who can help and they would like some extra help, ask them to put their speaker phone on.
- Check with the person that you understand what they are saying (e.g. 'Your head hurts, have I got that right?').
- Some individuals with autism have difficulty interpreting tone of voice, so do not rely on this alone when communicating a message.
- If you suspect that the caller is only answering questions with a 'yes' (for example) consider whether you need to ask the question in a different way.
- Consider whether the call should be handled by a more senior or clinical colleague.

Time out activity – consider the following scenario

David has a learning disability and had started to feel unwell, so he rang 999. During the call, David became anxious as he had never called 999 before. This made it difficult for him to understand some of the questions and remember his personal information. The call handler recognised that David was struggling and asked him whether he had any difficulties or disabilities that might make the call hard for him. David clarified that he had a learning disability and remembered that he had a health passport which he could use to support him with the call. He also turned the radio off to reduce background distractions. The call handler asked David what she could do to make the call better for him; David asked her to speak clearly and explain any complicated words. The call handler then checked whether David understood each question and gave him longer to answer.

What techniques did the call handler use to help David?

Vulnerability and Learning Disabilities/Autism

People with learning disabilities and autism can be more vulnerable to harm due to their disability. As with other types of abuse, this harm could take the form of physical or mental abuse, financial abuse or sexual abuse.

People with learning disabilities and autism are also often victims of hate crimes. Disability hate crime is when a person is attacked, threatened or verbally abused as a result of their disability, or perceived disability [Disability Rights UK, 2015]. Staggeringly, as many as 88% of people with learning disabilities have reported some form of bullying or harassment [Mencap, 2013]. There have been a number of tragic cases where people with learning disabilities have been murdered as a result of their disability.

As with any safeguarding concern, make sure you report it straight away in line with your organisational policies and procedures.

Summary

This chapter has defined learning disabilities and autism, described their causes and discussed some

key legislation. It has taken the approach that autism and learning disabilities can be present together as well as individually and aims to make the call handler aware that, while managing a call with people with learning disabilities and autism may present distinct challenges, there are ways to improve the caller's experience. The call handler should aim to make the call as easy as possible for the individual by adapting their communication style and being aware of individual needs to ensure the safe and effective management of the call.

References and Further Reading

Material in this chapter has been reproduced from: Richard Pilbery and Kris Lethbridge, *Ambulance Care Practice*, Bridgwater: Class Publishing (2016), with kind permission from the authors.

Department of Health (2001). *Valuing people*. Available at: https://www.gov.uk/government/uploads/system/ uploads /attachment_data/file/250877/5086.pdf (last accessed 14 June 2015).

Department of Health (2015). *Working together to safeguard children*. Available at: https://www.gov.uk/ government/publications/working-together-to-safeguard-children--2 (Accessed 7 June 2018).

Disability Rights UK (2012). *Disability Rights UK Factsheet F20*. Available: https://www.disabilityrightsuk.org/ how-we-can-help/independent-living/stop-disability-hate-crime (last accessed: 8 June 2018)

Disability Rights UK (2012). *Disability Rights UK Factsheet F20*. Available: https://www.disabilityrightsuk.org/ how-we-can-help/independent-living/stop-disability-hate-crime (last accessed: 8 June 2018).

Holland, K. (2011). *Factsheet: Learning Disabilities*. Available at: http://www.bild.org.uk/EasySiteWeb/GatewayLink. aspx?alld=2522 (last accessed 14 June 2015).

Medical Research Council (2001). *MRC Review of Autism Research: Causes and Epidemiology*. Available at: https://mrc.ukri.org/publications/browse/autism-research-review/ (last accessed 9 April 2018).

Mencap (2013). *Four things you probably didn't know about disability hate crime*. Available at: https://www. mencap.org.uk/blog/four-things-you-probably-didnt-know-aboutdisability-hate-crime (Accessed 6 December 2015).

Mencap (2015). *About learning disability*. Available at: https://www.mencap.org.uk/about-learning-disability/ about-learning-disability (last accessed 14 June 2015).

National Autistic Society (2018). *Autism facts and history*. Available at: http://www.autism.org.uk/about/ what-is/myths-facts-stats.aspx (last accessed 0 April 2018).

NHS Choices (2013). *What is a learning disability?* Available at: http://www.nhs.uk/Livewell/Childrenwithalearning disability/Pages/Whatislearningdisability.aspx (last accessed 14 June 2015).

NHS Digital (2016). *Adult Psychiatric Morbidity Survey: Survey of Mental Health and Wellbeing, England, 2014.* Available: http://digital.nhs.uk/catalogue/PUB21748 (last accessed 8 June 2018)

NSPCC (2015). *How safe are our children?* Available at: https://www.nspcc.org.uk/globalassets/documents/ research-reports/how-safe-children-2015-report.pdf (last accessed 20 June 2018).

Pilbery, R. and Lethbridge, K. (2016). *Ambulance Care Practice*. Bridgwater: Class Publishing.

Westminster Autism Commission (2016). *A Spectrum of Obstacles*. Available at: https://westminsterautism commission.files.wordpress.com/2016/03/ar1011_ ncg-autism-report-july-2016.pdf (last accessed 10 April 2018).

Chapter 9: Anatomy, Physiology and Pathophysiology: A Systems Approach

Learning Objectives

By the end of this chapter you will be able to:

- Describe the priorities of ruling out life-threatening situations over the telephone
- State examples of how ABCs may be compromised
- Describe how the body deals with illness and injury
- State the basic principles of how cells make up all the systems of the body
- Explain the basic functions of each body system
- Describe some of the examples of what can go wrong with each body system.

Life-threatening Situations

The priority when conducting a telephone assessment is to establish whether the patient's condition is immediately life-threatening. Cells need a constant supply of oxygen to survive, especially brain cells, which begin to die after 3–5 minutes with no oxygen. Therefore, we need to quickly establish whether oxygen is being circulated around the body.

To keep the body supplied with oxygen three things are essential:

A (AIRWAY): a clear airway through which air, containing oxygen, can enter

B (BREATHING): air enters the lungs where oxygen passes into the blood

C (CIRCULATION): a pumping heart and enough blood to carry oxygen to the body.

This is why we use the term assessing a person's **ABCs**.

> ## Time out activity – recognising serious problems associated with ABCs
>
> What phrases might a caller use to indicate that there is a serious problem with someone's airway, breathing or circulation? Here are a couple of examples to get you thinking.
>
> 'He's not breathing' or 'She's collapsed on the floor and looks a funny colour.'

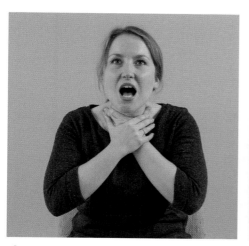

Figure 9.1(a) A patient who is choking

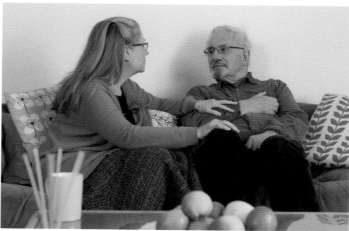

Figure 9.1(b) A patient experiencing chest pain

If you establish that someone's life is in immediate danger the priority is to get an ambulance to them as quickly as possible. Remember, it is not your job to try and diagnose what the problem is. However, having some knowledge of potential causes can help us understand the questions we are asking and correctly interpret the information callers provide. So let's consider some causes.

Airway

Anything blocking the passage of air through the airways into the lungs can stop oxygen reaching the body. Reasons for this include:

- Choking
- Unconsciousness: when a person is unconscious the tongue may flop back and prevent air entering the airway.

Breathing

We already know that a blocked airway stops a person breathing, but many other things can do this such as a heart attack, an injury to the chest or head, drowning, a severe allergy, or poisoning by drugs or toxic gases. A person who stops breathing will become unconscious. Their chest will not be moving, there will be no breath sounds and their skin may look very pale, grey or blue.

Circulation

The body needs a pumping heart, together with enough blood to transport oxygen. Shock is a life-threatening condition that occurs when the cardiovascular system (consisting of the heart, blood and blood vessels) fails and is unable to circulate adequate amounts of oxygen around the body. This can quickly lead to death. Shock in this context does not mean someone who is startled or has had a fright. When assessing shock over the telephone, the key features to bear in mind are:

- The person will be collapsed meaning that they are very weak and unable to stand. They may also be completely unconscious.
- Someone who is experiencing true clinical shock will have cold skin, which can also feel clammy or wet. Patients may describe this clamminess in different ways, such as 'sweatiness' or 'wetness'. Stimulation of the sweat glands by the nervous system occurs in response to this crisis situation, which causes this (cold) sweating. Their skin will also be much paler than usual or even grey or blue because the body diverts blood from the skin to more essential organs.

Causes of Shock

These include:

- Severe blood loss due to excessive bleeding from a wound or internal bleeding from an organ like the liver or from a blood vessel damaged by a bone fracture.
- Heavy fluid loss (e.g. due to vomiting, diarrhoea or through severe burns).
- Failure of the heart to pump properly (e.g. due to a heart attack).
- Anaphylaxis (life-threatening allergic reaction).
- Other causes such as severe infections, low blood sugar or a lack of certain hormones.

Basic Life Support

If a person's ABCs are compromised for any reason, they may well need the intervention of basic life support (BLS) with cardiopulmonary resuscitation (CPR). Everyone will have different levels of experience in basic life support, from no knowledge at all, to full and in-depth training. However, the clinical decision support system (CDSS) have instructions to enable you to instruct someone in CPR prior to help arriving.

If a person requires basic life support, speed is of the essence. If an automatic external defibrillator

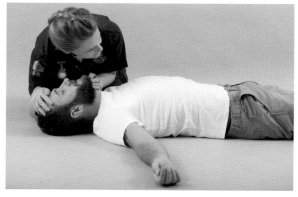

Figure 9.2 A paramedic on scene checking for breathing

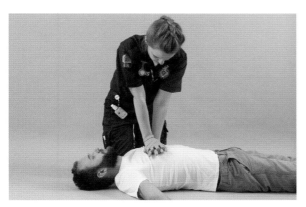

Figure 9.3 Providing basic life support

(AED) is available, this is another way of potentially increasing the patient's chance of survival. An AED is a portable electronic device that automatically diagnoses certain types of life-threatening problems with the heart's rhythm and can treat these with an electric shock.

The evidence to support early defibrillation is very clear: the delay from when a person collapses to the delivery of the first shock is the single most important determining factor in survival. If defibrillation occurs quickly, survival rates as high as 75% have been reported.

AEDs are simple to use and are now found in many public places. In order to make them highly visible, AEDs often are brightly coloured and mounted in protective cases near the entrance of a building. Most AEDs have spoken prompts and some may also have visual displays to instruct the user. When turned on or opened, the AED guides the user through the process of using it. Once a shock is given the machine will analyse the heart rhythm and either instruct CPR to be given or administer another shock.

Most patients who have a cardiac arrest will stop breathing immediately. However in the first few minutes after a sudden cardiac arrest, about 40% of patients may be barely breathing, or taking infrequent, noisy, gasps. This is called 'agonal breathing' and should not be confused with normal breathing. Agonal breathing is an abnormal breathing pattern where there are slow, sometimes noisy, irregular breaths that usually occur about every 10–15 seconds. This type of breathing can continue for several minutes after the heart has stopped beating.

The person with agonal breathing might be described as 'gasping', 'snorting', 'gurgling' or 'making funny noises'. They will be collapsed and unconscious. If there is doubt as to whether an unconscious person is breathing normally it should be assumed that they are not. Many public places have AEDs (public access defibrillators) and the ambulance service will be responsible for providing access codes for those that are kept in a locked cabinet.

The Body's Response to Illness and Injury

Within this section we will explore how the body responds to illness and injury. It is important to be able to distinguish between illness and injury as the reason for a person's call as these are assessed and dealt with in a different way. Let's look at each of these in turn.

Illnesses

Illness is very common. Everyone is ill from time to time and these illnesses have a multitude of different causes. Viral and bacterial infections are the most common causes of illness. When viruses or bacteria invade the body and either grow or reproduce, they usually produce side effects that cause illness and damage. For example, the polio virus releases poisons that destroy nerve cells, often leading to paralysis. Also, as we will discover in the section on the immune system, our body works hard to try and fight off the invading germs and this immune response also produces side effects such as swollen glands, a high temperature, swelling or a discharge which makes us feel unwell.

When an organ becomes weak or damaged it can cause illness (e.g. heart disease). Alternatively, illness can occur when cells start to grow abnormally. Normal body cells grow and die in an orderly way. Cancer develops when cells in parts of the body grow rapidly in an uncontrolled way and replace normal tissue.

Illness can also be the result of faulty genes. Genes carry inherited information about how to make the proteins we need to grow, function properly and stay healthy. An example of an illness caused by faulty genes is haemophilia, where the blood doesn't clot properly. Blood clotting is

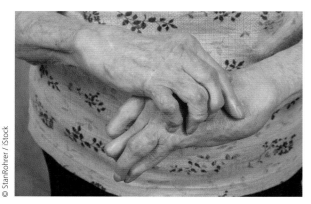

© StanRohrer / iStock

Figure 9.4 Arthritic hands

essential after an injury to stop excessive blood loss. The faulty genes in people with haemophilia mean that they don't have enough special clotting proteins and are at great risk if they cut or bruise themselves.

Another example of a genetic condition is sickle cell disease. This is an inherited disorder that affects red blood cells. Normal red blood cells are shaped a bit like a doughnut, and because of their structure they can move through small blood vessels to deliver oxygen. Sickle red blood cells are hard, sticky and misshapen like a 'sickle' which means when they try to travel through small vessels they block the flow of blood and break apart. This can cause pain, damage and a low red blood cell count. Most people with this disorder will know they have it and might have special instructions about how to manage their condition. It is important to listen to what they say about their condition and if ever you are in doubt about how to manage something, make sure you get some clinical advice.

Cells in the immune system can also lose their ability to tell the difference between normal tissue and germs that may be causing problems. When this happens the immune system can attack the person's own body. An example of this is rheumatoid arthritis, shown in Figure 9.4, where the normal tissue in a person's joints is attacked by a process normally designed to protect the body.

Some illnesses start suddenly and are short lived. These illnesses, where the person recovers

relatively quickly, are described as 'acute'. Other illnesses, however, persist over a long period of time. The symptoms often appear gradually, get worse despite treatment or change very slowly. These conditions are termed 'chronic'. It is important to be able to assess whether the symptoms a person describes are new and therefore part of an acute disorder, or long-standing and part of a more chronic condition.

People with potentially life-threatening chronic conditions such as diabetes will often wear a medical alert bracelet or pendant (often called a MedicAlert®), which identifies their condition and helps healthcare professionals to treat them appropriately.

Injuries

Some of your callers will be contacting your service for help in dealing with an injury. An injury (sometimes referred to as a trauma) is when the body has suffered a physical injury. Injuries can either be penetrating, where there is a break in the skin or other body surface (e.g. an accidental cut or a deliberate stab wound) or blunt where the skin or other body surface has not been broken but damage has still occurred (e.g. a bruise).

Blunt and penetrating injuries often need to be dealt with differently. For example, with a penetrating injury there is likely to be visible bleeding, and an increased risk of germs getting in and causing infection. With a blunt injury there will be no visible external bleeding, but there may be swelling, bruising and internal damage to joints, muscles or internal organs.

These types of injury are especially common in children and are the most common cause of death in this age group. In all age groups, injuries can range from life-threatening to very minor.

When someone has experienced an injury, one of your tasks will be to try and find out how serious it is likely to be. Remember, the purpose of telephone triage is not to offer the caller a diagnosis, but to be able to direct them to the most appropriate care in the most appropriate timeframe. Often in very serious situations, it quickly becomes obvious how severe the injury is due to the description of the person's problem

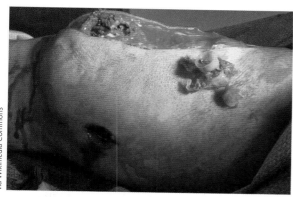

Figure 9.5 Gunshot wound

(e.g. where the person is unconscious, not breathing or where there is blood spurting from a wound). In this situation we don't need to ask any more questions to be able to advise what needs to be done, how quickly it needs to happen and where they need to be taken.

At other times we make an educated assumption that the injury is likely to have very serious and possibly life-threatening consequences because of the way it was caused. Examples include:

- Serious burns (e.g. those involving a large surface area or a burn caused by inhaling hot gases)
- Serious wounds (e.g. wounds caused by a gunshot or stabbing – see Figure 9.5)
- Limb amputation
- Injuries caused by road traffic collisions
- Near drowning
- A fall from a height, which can cause injury to several parts of the body.

These are just some examples, not an exhaustive list. Your clinical decision support system (CDSS) will provide questions to enable you to pick up serious injuries, as well as more minor ones.

How the Body Heals Itself

The body is usually remarkably good at coping with illness and injury and there are different ways in which this works. Blood clotting and fever are examples of this and are discussed in this section.

Blood Clotting and Inflammation

Platelets are structures within the blood that are important for blood clotting. When there is damage to part of the body a chemical protein inside platelets causes them to become sticky. This helps them combine with other substances to form a clot, which basically plugs the hole and stops bleeding. The clot later dries out to become a scab that helps to stop germs entering and then new skin forms underneath.

Some people have faulty blood clotting mechanisms. The problem may have a wide range of causes from faulty genes (e.g. haemophilia) to particular medicines (e.g. warfarin). Some disorders mean that the blood can be too prone to clotting whereas others can mean that the blood doesn't clot properly. If someone has blood which clots too easily they may need an anti-coagulant drug which makes the blood less prone to clotting. If someone has been injured it can take longer for the bleeding to stop if they have a problem with clotting or they take anticoagulant drugs, meaning that more urgent treatment may be required.

The inflammatory response occurs when tissues are injured (e.g. by germs, injury, heat or poisons). Chemicals are released by the damaged tissue and these cause blood vessels to leak fluid into the tissues, causing swelling. One of these chemicals, histamine, helps to isolate the harmful substance. The chemicals also attract white blood cells that 'eat' germs, dead or damaged cells. All of this activity often makes the area swell up and become warmer than the surrounding area. As the body continues to fight the problem and deal with the damage, pus is often formed. (This is a collection of dead tissue, dead bacteria and white blood cells.) This pus can then form a swelling under the skin (a boil or an abscess) which usually finds an opening on the surface and discharges onto the skin. As everything settles down, the swelling goes and the inflammation in the area disappears.

Fever

Fever – a raised temperature – occurs when the body's thermostat inside the brain (located in the hypothalamus) raises body temperature above its normal level. This thermostat knows what temperature the body should be (usually around

37°C) and sends signals around the body to maintain this.

Sometimes the thermostat will reset the body to a higher temperature in response to infection or inflammation. It is thought that this is the body's way of fighting the germs that cause infection. Fever is not an illness but a sign of an underlying problem. The fever itself is rarely harmful but it can make a person feel uncomfortable. Along with the rise in body temperature, symptoms of a fever may include sweating, chills and skin that is hot to touch. A temperature is also often associated with aches and pains and a headache, and the person may have a flushed face and occasionally violent shivering if the temperature is very high or rises very quickly. The violent shivering which occurs with especially high fevers is called a rigor. Muscles at work generate a lot of heat, which is why we get hot and go red when we exercise.

Rigor happens when the body's muscles are shivering very hard in an attempt to raise body temperature to the new level set by the thermostat. These aren't normal shivers and may be so strong the person might even notice their bed or chair shake when the rigor comes on. Until the body reaches the temperature the thermostat requires, the person may feel cold. This is why people with a fever sometimes wrap themselves up in lots of clothes or blankets.

Antibiotics

Sometimes the body needs help to heal itself, for example, if someone develops a serious bacterial infection.

Antibiotics are important and sometimes life-saving medicines used to treat bacterial illnesses. Although they kill bacteria they have no effect on human cells or viruses. Viruses don't have the same 'machinery' as bacteria. As it is this machinery that is targeted by antibiotics, they are useless in dealing with viruses.

A problem with antibiotics is that they lose effectiveness if they are overused. Antibiotics normally kill their target bacteria in a week or 10 days but the patient usually feels better in a day or two because the majority of bacteria are killed quickly. However, sometimes one of the bacteria offspring develops resistance and is able to survive the antibiotic treatment. This is particularly likely if people stop the treatment before the end of the course. If this strand of bacteria then multiplies the

whole disease changes. If the new strain of the disease then infects other people, the old antibiotic has no effect. That is what is known as antibiotic resistance. It is vital that antibiotics are only used when absolutely necessary to reduce the risk of resistance and it is essential that people take the whole course of treatment. Another problem with antibiotics is that they may also kill the good bacteria in our bodies that help us stay healthy. This is how we sometimes get diarrhoea after antibiotic treatment for a severe sore throat or chest infection.

The Body's Building Blocks

Before we consider each system of the body we need to consider how its structure is made up. The basic building block of every living thing is the cell. Cells are extremely complex, come in different forms, and have lots of different functions. A group of similar cells gathered together is called tissue. Bone, muscle and fat are all different types of tissue. Different kinds of tissue working together in the same place may form an organ, such as the heart, lungs, skin and brain. Several organs can work together in a system, such as the digestive, reproductive, respiratory and nervous systems.

If you want to understand how the body works, you need a basic understanding of cells. Everything from reproduction to repairing a broken bone happens at cell level. All of the work done inside a cell is reliant on enzymes; these are substances that allow the cell to carry out chemical reactions very quickly. The life of a cell is dependent on a rich soup of enzymes that float within it. Many different medicines or poisons work by affecting this soup in some way. For example the antibiotic penicillin can prevent a bacterium from building cell walls. Because bacterial cell walls and human cell walls are very different, the penicillin interferes with the bacteria but does not affect the human cells.

Cells grow by division. One cell doubles by dividing into two, these two cells become four and so on. In adults, cells normally only divide to replace those that have died (e.g. through injury, illness or as part of renewing things like our hair and skin). Cell growth is normally carefully controlled, but sometimes cells suddenly start to grow rapidly in an uncontrolled way. This is what happens when a person develops cancer. The cancer cells continue to divide and form a lump. New lumps in the body are often called tumours. Some tumours may grow, but do not spread to other parts of the body. These tumours are described as 'benign' and may not need any treatment. However some tumours do spread. This type of tumour is called 'malignant' and is usually referred to as 'cancer'.

In addition to surgery, cancer is often treated by radiotherapy and/or chemotherapy. Chemotherapy is a drug treatment which is used to try and kill cancer cells or stop them spreading. Because chemotherapy drugs are absorbed into the bloodstream, they travel around the body and can attack cancer cells regardless of where they find them. Radiotherapy uses x-rays (radiation) to destroy cancer cells. It can only be given to small areas of the body or it will cause damage to many healthy cells.

The cancer itself as well as some treatments can make people especially prone to infection. If the person's symptoms suggested that they might have an infection, for example they had a high temperature or felt unwell, then it is especially important that they receive prompt treatment. Also as we have discovered, cancer can spread to other parts of the body and can also reoccur after it has been treated. A new symptom that starts in someone with a history of cancer needs to be checked in case it is related to the cancer or its treatment. So any symptoms which suggest this might be the case require prompt assessment by the person's own GP.

Systems of the Body

The Cardiovascular System

The cardiovascular system consists of the heart (cardio) and blood and blood vessels (vascular). The heart lies behind the rib cage between the lungs. This is the pump that moves blood around the system. A typical body has about 4–5 litres of blood that is carried round the body in three main types of blood vessels: arteries, veins and capillaries. The arteries carry the blood away from the heart and veins bring it back. The capillaries are the vital bits in the middle where the oxygen in the blood and the food for the body tissues is delivered. It is in these tiny blood vessels that the blood also collects the waste products from the cells and takes it away for 'recycling' or disposal.

How does oxygen get into the blood? When you breathe in, air is sucked into your lungs. As well as

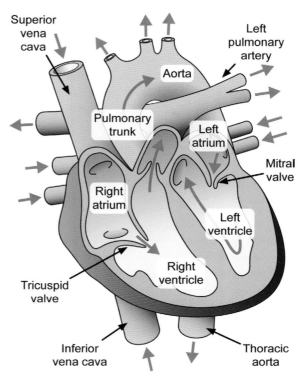

Figure 9.6 Chambers of the heart and related anatomy

going round the rest of the body, blood is pumped from the heart to the lungs, to collect the vital oxygen from the air you have inhaled. This oxygen-rich blood travels back to the heart before it is pumped through arteries which gradually divide into the tiny capillaries. In the capillaries, the nutrients from our food and oxygen from the air we breathe are released into all the cells in the body. Carbon dioxide is one of the main waste products from cells, and in the capillaries this is swapped with the oxygen in the fresh blood arriving from the heart. The oxygen-depleted blood, with its waste carbon dioxide, is then carried back to the heart, and the cycle begins again.

The largest artery in the body, connected directly to the heart, is the aorta. Because the heart is a pump and arteries carry blood directly away from the heart, blood in them travels in spurts or surges with every heartbeat. If we count the number of these surges or spurts in an artery we call it taking the pulse rate. When a person has a wound that has cut through an artery, the blood will spurt out with every heartbeat. Blood loss from an artery is therefore very rapid as the blood is being pumped by the heart under significant pressure. Remember the veins? These are the blood vessels carrying blood back to the heart. If the arteries are like fast flowing rivers, the veins are more like slow moving canals collecting blood from the capillaries. Unlike arteries, the veins are not under pressure and do not have a pulse. So while blood from a cut artery will spurt out and large amounts will be lost very quickly, bleeding from a cut vein tends to be more of an ooze.

When someone loses blood, various complex mechanisms in the body come into effect, which help to try and make up or 'compensate' for the blood lost. This blood loss can be external (e.g. bleeding from a wound) or it may be internal (e.g. bleeding from a stomach ulcer). If only a small amount of blood is lost, either internally or externally, the body needs to do very little to compensate. However, if a larger amount is lost, the body will need to do more to try and ensure adequate circulation around the body (e.g. diverting blood away from the skin to major organs such as the brain). If a large volume of blood is lost in a short period of time, the body may find it impossible to compensate and the situation may become life-threatening.

There are two vital statistics that are used to assess the immediate health of your heart: blood pressure and pulse. These fluctuate as the condition of your heart changes. Your pulse is taken by pressing one of several pulse points. This is where the arteries are close enough to the surface of the skin for the 'spurts' that we talked about earlier to be felt. This makes it possible to measure heart rate by counting contractions of the artery. Blood pressure is the force of blood against the artery walls. It is recorded as two numbers: the systolic pressure (as the heart beats) over the diastolic pressure (as the heart relaxes between beats). This second measurement reflects how much the small arteries in the body are resisting the flow of blood into them. Some people have machines at home to help them monitor their blood pressure. If someone has called about concerns with their blood pressure but is not complaining of any particular symptom, seek advice from a clinician.

The heart is an amazing organ, which in an average lifetime beats more than two-and-a-half billion times without ever pausing to rest. Made

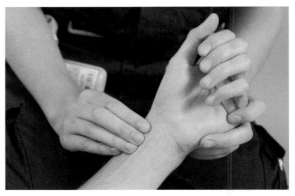

Figure 9.7 A paramedic measuring someone's pulse

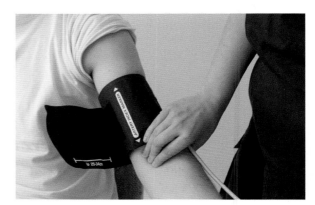

Figure 9.8 Blood pressure measurement

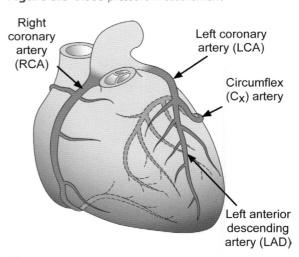

Figure 9.9 Coronary artery anatomy

of muscle, the heart contracts about 70 or so times a minute at rest. Have you ever noticed that your heart speeds up even when you are not exercising? When you are nervous, the hormone adrenaline is secreted in tiny amounts by the adrenal glands (situated just above the kidneys). It raises your heart rate immediately, preparing you for action. This is what is known as the 'fight or flight' response. Caffeine and other factors can also affect heart rate and can cause palpitations.

Time out activity – recognising palpitations over the telephone

Think about a time when you have been exercising very hard and could feel your heart beating. What words would you use to describe the way it felt?

Now think about a time when you were incredibly excited or scared and could feel your heart beating. What words would you use to describe the way it felt?

These are likely to be some of the words and phrases callers use to describe palpitations.

You may receive calls from people suffering from palpitations. This term is used when someone experiences the sensation of their heart beating irregularly or more rapidly or forcefully than it should. There are many causes ranging from the very serious to those which are more minor. People use different ways to describe the feeling and not everyone knows what the term 'palpitations' means, so they may use terms like 'thudding', 'racing', 'fluttering' or 'missing a beat'. You've probably come up with some others.

Time out activity – symptoms of coronary heart disease

Although the heart is continually filled with blood, this blood does not provide it with oxygen. The blood supply that provides oxygen and nutrients to the heart is provided by blood vessels that wrap around the outside of the heart. Coronary heart disease happens when these arteries become narrowed. This restricts the supply of blood and oxygen to the heart itself, particularly when the demands of the heart muscle increase (e.g. during exercise). Based on what you know about the heart and what it does, what type of symptoms do you think a person with coronary heart disease might have?

Remember, the purpose of this activity is not to enable you to tell when a person has heart disease – this is the job of specialist doctors – but is to help you become familiar with the range of symptoms that people may describe over the phone.

What Can Go Wrong?

Angina

The main symptom of coronary heart disease is angina. This is caused by a lack of oxygen to the heart muscle because of poor blood flow. People may describe angina as a feeling of heaviness, pressure, tightness or pain in the centre of the chest that may either spread to or just affect the arms, neck, jaw, face, back or abdomen. Angina sufferers are most likely to experience it during exertion (for instance when climbing stairs or playing sports). It can also come on in cold weather, after a heavy meal or during times of stress. Usually it goes away once the person rests or takes their angina medication. Although all chest pain needs to be taken seriously, not every type of chest pain is angina. Angina is a diagnosis given by doctors after carrying out certain assessments or tests. A person with angina will recognise their pain and will know their normal treatment and how long it normally takes to work. If a person's angina does not go away when they take their medication or if it comes back after a short period of time when the person is just resting, there is a serious risk of a heart attack.

Unfortunately, for many people, a heart attack is the first sign that something is wrong. A heart attack occurs when the blood supply to part of the heart muscle is cut off, usually because of a blood clot. The pain of a heart attack is often severe but may also be mistaken for bad indigestion. The main symptoms are:

- Persistent chest pain (often described as crushing, tight, a feeling of heaviness, pressure or pain in the centre of the chest) which may spread to the arms, neck, jaw, face, back or abdomen (or may just affect these areas in isolation). Unlike angina, this doesn't go away when the person rests
- Breathlessness or gasping for air
- Faintness, dizziness or collapse
- Sweating
- A sense that something is seriously wrong ('impending sense of doom')
- Nausea
- Grey/pale skin and blue tinge around the mouth
- A rapid, weak or irregular pulse.

Heart Attack

If the blood supply is cut off for a long time, the muscle cells die due to a lack of oxygen. If enough cells die, the heart cannot function and stops beating altogether. Often, however, only a small part of heart muscle dies and the rest of the heart muscle compensates so the person recovers. This is called a myocardial infarction. However, in discussing this with patients you should use the term 'heart attack'. Drugs such as aspirin and medications that dissolve the clot are used to limit the amount of muscle damage. The quicker these are given, the more likely it is that the heart will recover.

Aortic Aneurysm

Arteries have thick, elastic walls to enable them to withstand normal blood pressure. However, sometimes these become weakened making them less able to withstand this pressure. An aneurysm is a bulging, weakened area in an artery wall. The force of blood pushing against a damaged area can cause an aneurysm. The bulge can be small and spherical, like a berry, or it can be larger and more balloon-like. Aneurysms can occur in any artery, but they are most common in the aorta and the arteries in the brain. Aortic aneurysms can develop anywhere along its length, but abdominal aortic aneurysms (AAA's) are by far the most common. Aneurysms that occur in the part of aorta that runs through the chest are called thoracic aortic aneurysms.

The most common cause of aortic aneurysm is atherosclerosis. This is where fatty deposits are laid down in the walls of arteries making them weaker. Risk factors for atherosclerosis include smoking, high blood pressure, high cholesterol, obesity and a family history of cardiovascular disease. There is also a familiar tendency to developing aortic aneurysms. Individuals with a close relative who have an aortic aneurysm have a higher risk of developing one themselves.

Certain diseases can also weaken the layers of the aortic wall and increase the risk of aortic aneurysms. These include genetic conditions such as Marfan syndrome, which affects the body's connective tissues. Age and gender also play a part. As a person ages the risk of developing an aneurysm increases and they are much more common in men than women.

Most aortic aneurysms don't cause symptoms so many people don't even know they have one. In fact most are diagnosed during tests performed for other reasons. People will be aware if they have been diagnosed with an aneurysm.

Like any balloon which gets bigger, there is a danger that it will burst. If an aortic aneurysm dissects or ruptures (bursts), a very large amount of blood can be lost from the circulation very quickly. This internal bleeding deprives essential organs of blood which, if not treated promptly, can lead to death.

Common symptoms of aortic rupture or dissection include:

- Shock, as so much blood is lost very quickly. The person may be cold, grey and sweaty.
- Extreme, constant and sudden pain, often described as ripping and tearing. It can occur in the chest, back, abdomen or flank and may radiate to other areas (e.g. the groin, buttocks, arms or legs).
- Nausea or vomiting.
- In some cases, little or no pain but a sense that something is very wrong.

The Nervous System

The nervous system is a highly complex system responsible for controlling the processes of the body. There are two main parts: the central nervous system consisting of the brain and spinal cord, and the peripheral nervous system consisting of the nerves which connect the central nervous system to the rest of the body. Additionally, the autonomic (involuntary) nervous system controls body functions such as digestion and breathing.

The brain is a very complex organ made up of billions of cells. It is wrinkled and has the consistency of blancmange. It is injured by even very slight pressure so needs to be well protected. This protection consists of:

- Three tough membranes called meninges which surround the brain.
- A clear fluid between the brain and meninges called cerebrospinal fluid. This cushions the brain, provides it with energy and protects it against infection.
- The bony case of the skull.

Time out activity – calls about problems associated with the nervous system

Any telephone triage service is likely to receive a significant amount of calls regarding signs and symptoms associated with the nervous system. Spend a short while thinking through some examples of this type of call.

What Can Go Wrong?

Levels of Consciousness

The brain is the source of consciousness, speech, thought and memory. When fully conscious we are alert and aware of what is going on around us. When a person is unconscious it is impossible to rouse (wake) them. When consciousness is impaired, basic survival mechanisms such as the ability to keep the airway open may not function, because of a lack of muscle control which allows the tongue to fall back, blocking the airway. When this happens, breathing becomes laboured and noisy or may become impossible. When we talked about the heart we focused on how vital it was that oxygen was pumped to the tissues. If the airway is blocked and oxygen can't be taken in, the blood cannot carry it and cells of the body will start to die. Therefore, the priority with any unconscious person is to establish that their airway is open.

There is no absolute divide between consciousness and unconsciousness. Impaired consciousness is the term used to describe a situation where a person is anything less than fully conscious. People with impaired consciousness may display signs such as being uncoordinated, drowsy, confused, slow to respond or have difficulty speaking. You will find questions within the NHS Pathways system designed to assess such situations.

You may receive calls about people who have experienced or who are currently experiencing a fit (also called a seizure or convulsion). Fits usually consist of involuntary spasms of many muscles in the body caused by a disturbance in the brain's electrical activity. They often result in loss or impairment of consciousness, so it is vital that the person's airway is protected. A common example is epilepsy. If a person suffers from epilepsy they may have treatment which can be administered into the rectum during a fit. Other causes of fits include a high fever, head injury, infections affecting the central nervous system, lack of oxygen or glucose to the brain and poisoning.

People can get distinctive feelings or warning signs that a seizure is on its way, known as auras. These will differ from person to person, but can include: feeling that the outside world has suddenly become unreal or dreamlike; stopping talking in

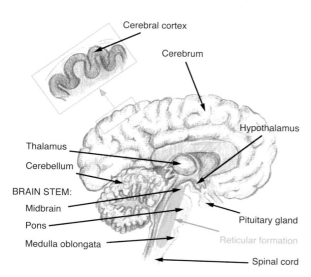

Figure 9.10 Brain

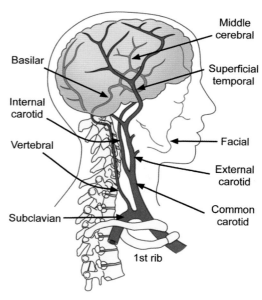

Figure 9.11 Brain and spinal cord

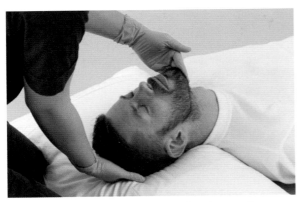

Figure 9.12 Paramedic opening the airway of an unconscious patient

the middle of a sentence or appearing to drift off. Although this warning cannot prevent the seizure, it can allow people around them to ensure they are in a safe place. Patients in the early stages of a cardiac arrest may display seizure-like episodes so when someone describes a patient having a fit or seizure it is vital to carefully assess whether they are actually breathing.

Dizziness is a feeling of unsteadiness or light headedness which you have probably experienced yourself at some time. Vertigo is something different. It is a specific medical term used to describe the sensation of spinning or having the room spinning about you. People find vertigo very disturbing and it is often associated with nausea and vomiting. Some of the most severe cases are caused by disorders of the balancing mechanisms in the inner ears and can cause the sufferer to fall over.

People may call about someone who has fainted. A faint is a sudden, temporary loss of consciousness. It is caused by a reduction in blood flow to the brain and, therefore, a lack of oxygen and glucose, causing the person to collapse and fall to the ground. If they are allowed to lie down, with their legs raised, blood flow to the brain is restored and recovery will be rapid. It is dangerous to keep a fainting person upright as it slows the return of normal circulation to the brain and prolongs the faint. In most cases of fainting, the person who has fainted regains consciousness within a minute or two. Anything longer is classed as a period of unconsciousness: the cause needs to be urgently established and the person treated as quickly as possible.

Meningitis and meningococcal septicaemia

Meningitis occurs when the meninges (i.e. the membranes that line the skull and enclose the brain and spinal cord) become inflamed. It can be caused by different organisms including bacteria and viruses. Common signs and symptoms are listed in Table 9.1.

What about a rash?

Some bacteria that cause meningitis can also cause sepsis, also often known as septicaemia or blood poisoning. As meningococcal bacteria multiply rapidly in the bloodstream, they begin to release endotoxins (poisons) from their outer coating. The body's natural defences have little effect on these poisons and eventually the blood vessels become damaged causing blood to leak into the tissues under the skin. The rash this produces may initially look like tiny pinpricks anywhere on the body but it can spread quickly to resemble bruises. It is more difficult to see on darker skin but may be more visible in paler areas, such as the mouth, palms, soles of feet, abdomen and under the eyelids.

This rash doesn't fade under pressure and you will have heard of the 'glass test' as a way of checking this. This is a very effective method of testing whether the rash fades under pressure, but can be difficult and time consuming to explain properly over the phone. It is also impossible to tell whether the test is being done correctly. For these reasons, callers should not be asked to perform the glass test, as this can waste valuable time and it is difficult to safely rely on results. However, if the caller has already done the glass test and the rash has not faded this information must be accepted.

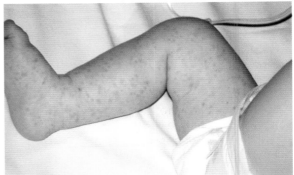

Figure 9.13 Septicaemic rash

Table 9.1 Common signs and symptoms of meningitis

Common signs and symptoms in babies and infants	Common signs and symptoms in children and adults
• Fever • Vomiting or refusing feeds • Very sleepy or reluctance to wake up • Becoming irritable and not wanting to be held • Ill appearance • Becoming floppy and unresponsive, or stiff with jerky movements • Unusual crying • Pale and blotchy skin • Bulging fontanelle – soft spot on baby's head • Very cold hands/feet	• A severe headache • Fever • Nausea and vomiting • Ill appearance • Altered mental state including confusion, delirium, drowsiness and impaired consciousness • Seizures or fits • Being unable to tolerate bright lights (photophobia) • A stiff neck – less common in young children • A rapid breathing rate • Severe muscle pain

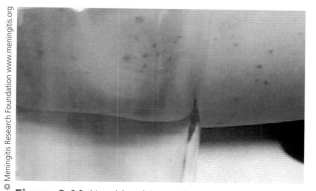

© Meningitis Research Foundation www.meningitis.org

Figure 9.14 Non-blanching rash

Meningitis and sepsis/septicaemia are not always easy to recognise. Many of the symptoms also occur with less serious (viral) illnesses. When the symptoms first begin, the person may not appear severely ill, parents may describe them as 'ill' or 'not their usual self' however these symptoms must always be taken seriously. As sepsis advances, it affects the whole body and can cause organ damage or failure: early treatment is therefore essential. We will talk about sepsis in more detail later, when we explore how the body copes with infection.

For more information go to: www.meningitisnow. org.

Damage to the Brain

A proportion of people calling your service will do so with signs and symptoms that may indicate injury to the brain. Although the brain is well protected, brain injuries can occur. Different parts of the brain do different things; the part of the brain injured will determine how the person is affected. The brain can be damaged by direct injuries such as a heavy blow during an assault or indirectly because the blood supply to a part of the brain has been interrupted. This is commonly known as a stroke. If brain cells do not get oxygen for 3–5 minutes, they begin to die. Stroke is a common cause of disability and death in the UK and, although it can occur at any age, most cases occur in people aged over 65.

Time out activity – signs and symptoms of a stroke

Strokes are relatively common and there has been a strong publicity campaign aimed at educating the public about its signs and symptoms. Many people are now aware of the symptoms and may call your service declaring that a person has suffered a stroke. Before reading on, spend a few moments thinking about what these symptoms might be.

Stroke

A stroke or 'cerebrovascular accident' (CVA) is always serious and can be life-threatening. The symptoms that occur following a stroke depend on the area of the brain affected and the extent of the damage.

Signs and symptoms of a stroke may include:

- Weakness of an arm or leg (or both) on the same side of the body ranging from total paralysis to mild clumsiness
- New facial weakness may also occur where one side of the face appears lopsided, and there may be drooling
- New numbness or tingling
- New confusion
- New difficulty speaking
- Headache, dizziness, unsteadiness, problems with vision, problems with swallowing
- Loss of consciousness or difficulty breathing in severe cases.

Just like heart attacks, if a stroke is caused by a blocked artery, it is now sometimes possible to clear the blockage and restore the circulation. It is vital that this is done as quickly as possible.

You may also hear people refer to a mini-stroke or 'TIA' (transient ischaemic attack). A TIA occurs when blood flow to part of the brain is blocked or reduced, usually by a clot, but just for a short period of time. The symptoms are the same as with a stroke, but they are more short-lived. However, TIA may be a warning sign that the person could have a stroke in the future.

Head Injuries

Because the brain acts as the body's 'command and control' centre, great caution needs to be exercised when dealing with head injuries. Guidelines have been developed by NICE (the National Institute for Health and Care Excellence) to help the NHS deal effectively with head injuries. Health professionals working in the NHS are expected to follow NICE's clinical guidelines.

Most head injuries assessed in an Emergency Department are mild and do not require the person to be admitted to hospital. However, serious head injuries can cause damage to the brain. Even mild head injuries can result in long-term problems (such as a persistent headache or problems concentrating). It is likely that the CDSS

in use within your organisation will have been built against the NICE head injury guidelines, so this will enable you to direct people to the most appropriate care.

Spinal Cord Injury

Another vital structure within the nervous system is the spinal cord. This is a collection of nerves running from the brain through a channel in the backbone or spine. The spinal cord carries nerve messages between the brain and the body. This allows the brain to control involuntary body processes, such as breathing and digestion, and to coordinate movement. There are nerves branching off from the spinal cord at different levels. This network of nerves is part of the peripheral nervous system. They carry information from the spinal cord to the rest of the body and from the body to the spinal cord, as nerve impulses.

Sitting deep within the bones of the spine, the spinal cord is well protected from injury. Like the brain, it is also protected by the meninges and cerebrospinal fluid. However, as we all know, spinal cord injuries do unfortunately occur and if the spinal cord is completely severed, the sections below the injury will be cut off from the brain. This means all nerves, and the parts of the body served by these nerves, will be disconnected from the brain and will stop functioning.

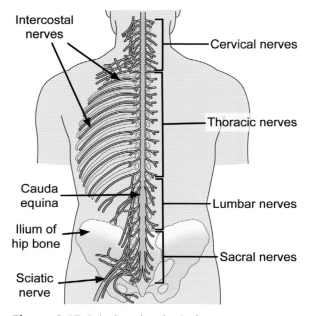

Figure 9.15 Spinal cord and spinal nerves

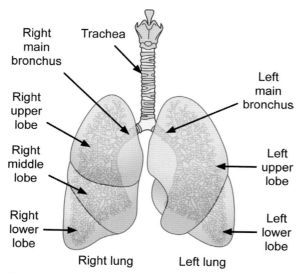

Right main bronchus

Trachea

Right upper lobe

Right middle lobe

Right lower lobe

Right lung

Left main bronchus

Left upper lobe

Left lower lobe

Left lung

Figure 9.16 The lower airway

The Respiratory System

All the cells in our body require oxygen. Without a constant supply of oxygen, cells would be unable to perform all their vital functions and we would die. As we discussed earlier, oxygen enters our respiratory system when we breathe in air. The respiratory system is situated in the chest and is responsible for the exchange of gases to and from our body.

So how does air enter the respiratory system? Well, we breathe in about 20 times a minute, with the help of a muscle called the diaphragm and other muscles in the chest and abdomen known as the intercostal muscles. The movement of these muscles results in pressure changes inside the lungs. When the diaphragm pulls down, it leaves more space for the lungs to expand and lowers the internal pressure. This results in air being sucked in which inflates the lungs. Think of the hand of a bicycle pump pulling air in and pushing it out as it moves up and down: the diaphragm does much the same in the chest.

When the diaphragm pushes up, the space inside the chest gets smaller and the pressure rises. This pushes air out of the lungs. When we breathe in, air enters the nose, where hairs and mucous filter and warm it. It continues down through the back of the throat into a tube called the trachea. This is also known as the airway. The trachea branches into two

tubes that enter the lungs. These divide into even smaller tubes, which end in air sacs called alveoli. Oxygen passes through the walls of the air sacs and enters the blood stream. At the same time, carbon dioxide passes into the lungs and is exhaled.

To keep things moving smoothly, the lungs are covered by two slippery layers of membrane called pleural membranes. Sometimes these membranes can become inflamed. This is usually due to infection. When this happens the membranes rub together producing a sharp pain, which is worse when the person breathes in or coughs.

The trachea is located at the front of the throat and the food tube or oesophagus is located at the back. This means that when we eat, food needs to move across the opening of our airway. To stop food entering, there is a small flap called the epiglottis across the opening of the trachea, which flops down to cover it when we swallow. We have all had the experience of something 'going down the wrong way' when we swallow something too quickly. This happens when the epiglottis doesn't have time to flop down and food or drink enters the airway. When this happens we cough automatically which usually clears it. However if the object is big enough and does not dislodge, it can completely block the airway. If this happens the person is said to be choking, which is an emergency situation. If the blockage partially obstructs the airway, the person will have difficulty breathing and speaking, will cough and be very distressed. A complete obstruction of the airway makes it impossible to speak, breathe or cough and the person will eventually lose consciousness if the blockage remains.

Assessing Breathing Difficulties over the Phone

Because a constant supply of oxygen is essential for life, any assessment of a person's health over the phone needs to quickly establish whether the person is able to breathe properly.

Everyone has experienced the feeling of being short of breath. Breathlessness is the feeling of having to work harder than normal to get air in and out of the lungs, like the feeling people get after running. When assessing breathlessness over the phone it is really important to find out how serious the problem is. This can be a little bit like putting pieces of a jigsaw together.

Time out activity – how people might describe breathing problems

Imagine that you have just run a race that involved running as fast as you could for as long as you could. What would your breathing be like? Spend some time thinking about the words or phrases you might use.

Now imagine a slightly different situation. Imagine you have just run down some stairs to answer a phone and that this has made you very slightly out of breath. What words or phrases might you use to describe this?

The previous activity may have identified that there are different degrees of breathing difficulty. It is important to be able to distinguish between these degrees of difficulty since different levels of breathing require a different response and different level of care. However there is no absolute dividing line between normal breathing and breathing difficulty. This can make assessing breathing problems over the telephone tricky. It may help to consider a continuum ranging from normal breathing to not breathing at all.

To be able to find out how severe the problem is, we need to be able to interpret the descriptions given by callers to describe breathing problems. It is really important to become familiar with the types of words and phrases people use and to become skilled at asking effective probing questions. Descriptions of breathing problems vary according to how bad the problem is. Some of the phrases that people might use to describe severe breathing problems include 'gasping for breath', 'unable to speak properly', 'wheezing badly' or 'croaking when they breathe'. These phrases are clearly different to the ones used to describe mild breathlessness such as 'a bit out of breath' or 'breathing more quickly than usual'. This does not mean that mild breathlessness is unimportant – all breathlessness needs to be taken seriously. However, severe breathlessness can be life-threatening, which means that further questions or pieces of the jigsaw are not needed before an ambulance is dispatched. If you talk to the patient themselves it is often much easier to assess their breathing, rather than trying to do this through a third party. You can actually hear how much difficulty the person is having, which is a big help in assessing the severity of the problem.

Common indicators of breathing difficulties are listed below to help you identify further key phrases or descriptions that may be used.

Common indicators of breathing difficulties include:

- Gasping for breath
- Unable to talk in full sentences
- Wheezing
- Noisy breathing
- Visibly struggling to breathe
- Supine position (lying on their back with face and torso pointing up)
- Blue tinge around mouth and nose (cyanosis)
- Rapid breathing
- May want to be outside (fresh air)
- Mild breathlessness.

Common indicators of breathing difficulties in infants may include:

- Chest and upper tummy being sucked in with every breath
- Head bobbing up and down when breathing
- Making a grunting noise with every breath
- Unable to cry properly.

Once we know that the person does not seem to be experiencing life-threatening breathlessness, there are other pieces of the jigsaw that need to be pieced together. This can include assessing how long the breathing problem has been present, how long it has taken to develop, whether it is getting

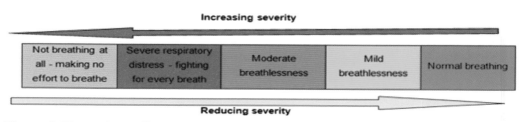

Figure 9.17 Breathing difficulty spectrum

Source: NHS Pathways Distance Learning Pack, NHS Digital

better or worse, whether this has happened before and whether there are any other symptoms. If these factors are important, then your system will provide questions for you to ask.

What Else Can Go Wrong?

There are many causes of breathing problems. The inhalation of gases (such as carbon monoxide), smoke or toxic vapours can affect breathing and prove fatal. Obstruction of the air passages of the nose, mouth or throat can cause problems, as well as problems affecting the airways and lungs, such as infection, severe allergies (see immune system section) and conditions such as asthma. Problems with other parts of the body such as the heart or kidneys can cause breathlessness, as can being very overweight. Emotional factors such as panic attacks can also cause shortness of breath.

Chest Infection

A chest infection is an infection of the lungs or large airways. Some chest infections are mild and clear up on their own, but others can be severe and life threatening. Anyone can have a chest infection, and they are common after having a cold or flu, especially in the autumn and winter.

The two main types of chest infection in adults are acute bronchitis and pneumonia. Acute bronchitis is an infection of the large bronchial tubes and is usually caused by a virus. Pneumonia, most commonly caused by bacteria, is an infection of the lungs in which the tiny sacs or alveoli become filled with fluid.

Common symptoms include:

- A chesty cough, often with green or yellow mucus
- Wheezing and shortness of breath
- Chest pain or discomfort
- A fever
- A headache, aching muscles and tiredness.

These symptoms can be unpleasant, but they usually get better on their own in about 7 to 10 days. The cough and mucus can last up to 3 weeks.

Asthma

There are a number of disorders that affect the respiratory system and one of the most common is asthma. This causes inflammation and narrowing of the airways. This makes it more difficult for air to pass through, resulting in the characteristic wheezing sound. Wheezing is a whistling or musical sound that comes from inside the chest when a person breathes. Aside from wheezing and shortness of breath, asthma can also cause a feeling of tightness in the chest or a cough. A person with asthma will usually be taking regular medication. How effectively the symptoms are controlled by the medication varies a lot between individuals. People with asthma, or their carer, can usually recognise when things are getting worse or out of control. It is important that rapidly worsening asthma is quickly assessed as it can be life-threatening.

Chronic Obstructive Pulmonary Disease (COPD)

Chronic obstructive pulmonary disease (COPD) is an umbrella term for a number of conditions where there is damage and inflammation to the lung. The symptoms of COPD include wheezing and breathlessness, chest tightness, a cough and increased phlegm production.

The main cause of COPD is smoking, but people with severe asthma can also develop the condition. Long-term exposure to pollution is another cause.

Chest Injuries

Injuries to the chest can also cause breathing problems. Both blunt and penetrating injuries can cause damage to the lung or pleural membranes. A penetrating wound can stop the chest moving air properly, just like if a bicycle pump had a hole in it. Penetrating chest wounds or blast injuries can also allow air to enter into the space between the pleural membranes (pleural cavity) causing a pneumothorax. This then puts pressure on the lung, which can cause it to collapse. This condition can also occur due to underlying lung disease. Signs and symptoms include sharp chest pain, breathlessness, blue discolouration to the skin, anxiety and sometimes a crackly feeling under the skin of the chest. The crackly feeling, which feels a bit like bubble-wrap being popped, is due to air from the lungs leaking under the skin.

Sometimes an injury can cause blood to collect in the pleural cavity. This is called a haemothorax and can stop the lung inflating properly. Characteristic signs and symptoms include chest pain, difficulty breathing, unequal chest expansion and, ultimately, shock. It can occasionally be caused by underlying medical conditions such as cancer or blood clotting disorders.

Drowning

Drowning, which is suffocation from being submerged in water is, by definition, fatal. However, some people rescued from the water may appear to be dead when they are actually still alive. On immersion in very cold water, the body responds by slowing the heart, reducing respiration and a dramatic change in circulation with blood going only to vital organs. If treated correctly, it is not unknown for such people to be saved. At the other end of the scale, a person may be involved in a near-drowning incident but may seem unharmed. However, if water has entered the lungs, it can cause irritation and swelling which may later prove fatal.

The Digestive System

The digestive system consists of a number of hollow organs that form a continuous passage from mouth to anus. This tube is also called the digestive tract. The purpose of this system is to break down food so that it can be used by cells for energy, growth and repair.

So, how does it do this? Well, after food is chewed and swallowed, it goes down the food pipe (the oesophagus) into the stomach. At the opening of the stomach there is a valve designed to seal it off. As food approaches the stomach, the valve opens and food enters. Here it is broken down by powerful stomach acids. Once it has become the consistency of thick soup it travels into the small intestine. In this part of the system, food is reduced to tiny particles and the nutrients are absorbed through the walls of the small intestine into the bloodstream. Anything that has not been absorbed into the bloodstream travels into the large intestine where any remaining nutrients and water can be absorbed by the body. Anything left over that the body cannot digest is stored in the rectum as the waste product, faeces, until this is expelled by a bowel movement. Movement through the system is controlled by muscles. These muscles can push food along the system or swill it around, to mix with digestive juices. So, for example, once we have swallowed some food, involuntary muscle movements in the oesophagus push it into our

stomach. Once in the stomach, food is moved backwards and forwards so that it mixes with the strong acid produced there, which helps with digestion.

What Can Go Wrong?

A significant proportion of the people that access the health service do so because of symptoms associated with the digestive system.

> ### Time out activity – calls associated with problems of the digestive system
>
> Before reading on, spend a few minutes thinking through possible reasons for people calling your service because of problems associated with the digestive system.

Abdominal Pain

A common symptom in patients making contact with telephone triage services is abdominal pain in both adults and children. There are many causes of abdominal pain, ranging from very serious to very minor. For example, a serious cause would include appendicitis, which is inflammation of the appendix; a condition which can become life-threatening if untreated. On the other end of the scale is something very minor like trapped wind, which can also cause abdominal pain. The degree of pain does not always indicate how serious the problem is, so a significant proportion of people complaining of abdominal pain need to be assessed by a doctor.

Not all pain in this area is caused by a condition affecting the digestive system. For example, the pain of a heart attack can be felt in the abdomen. Another example is the severe and sudden pain that is felt in the abdomen when the aorta (the main artery from the heart) splits. Sometimes the type of pain gives us some very useful clues as to how urgently the person requires further assessment. As with any other problem, assessing abdominal pain is like putting pieces of a jigsaw together. It is important to ask all the questions presented by your CDSS system in order to be able to provide the person with safe instructions.

Other common symptoms associated with this body system are vomiting and diarrhoea. Let's look at each of these in turn.

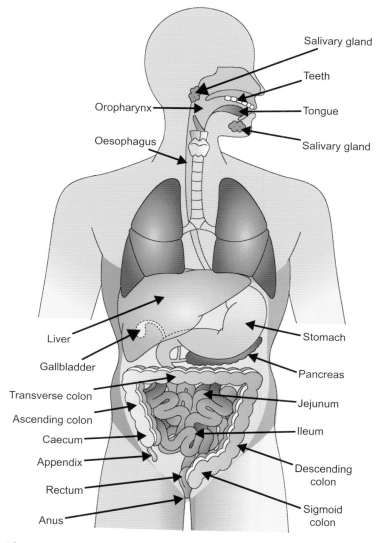

Figure 9.18 Overview of the digestive system

Vomiting

This has many different causes. Some of the more common are infections causes by viruses, bacteria and other bugs, excessive consumption of alcohol, morning sickness, motion sickness, inflammation of the stomach lining and reactions to medications. Less common causes include kidney disease, cancer and obstruction of the intestine, a head injury, diabetes and appendicitis.

Diarrhoea

This occurs when a person passes frequent loose or watery stools. As food passes through our system, water and any remaining nutrients are absorbed into the body through the walls of the large intestine. If this process is speeded up, less fluid, vitamins, minerals and salts are absorbed back into the body, resulting in these being passed in faeces. Like vomiting, diarrhoea has many causes, most of which are not serious.

Anything that irritates the intestine and speeds up the passage of food can cause diarrhoea. The most common cause is an infection caused by a virus, bacteria or other bug. Some people are sensitive to certain foods, which may lead to diarrhoea. Some medications, such as antibiotics and laxatives, may also cause the symptoms. Stress can lead to diarrhoea due to the effects of adrenaline, a hormone which speeds up body processes. These types of diarrhoea are usually short-lived but, when it persists, it can signal more serious illness.

Often a person will have diarrhoea and vomiting together. Because both produce a loss of fluid from the body, this can lead to dehydration more quickly than if the person is suffering from either symptom alone. Anything more than mild dehydration means the body lacks enough fluid to function properly. It is particularly dangerous in children and the elderly, and it must be treated promptly to avoid serious health problems.

A less common situation is where someone is experiencing bleeding from somewhere in their digestive system. This is more common in adults, but can occur in children. Symptoms depend on where the bleeding is coming from as well as how much and how quickly blood is being lost. Often there will be evidence of this blood within any vomited material or within the stool. However, the blood's appearance depends on where it is coming from. Blood lost from the upper digestive tract makes the stool appear black and like tar because the blood has travelled through most of the digestive tract and has been exposed to digestive juices. This is different to a normal motion that may simply be dark in colour. This is a very serious situation so it is important to ensure that the caller understands the question and that you interpret their answer correctly. Bleeding lower down in the digestive tract may make the stool look red or the person may pass blood straight into the toilet. Sometimes if a person experiences bleeding high up in the digestive tract they vomit or bring up blood. This may appear bright red or have lots of dark brown bits in it resembling soil or coffee-grounds because the blood reacts on contact with stomach acid. Vomiting blood needs urgent assessment as the bleeding can be severe and therefore life-threatening. A caller may not always recognise blood in vomit or stools so you may need to get them to describe it to you.

A stoma is a surgically created opening of the bowel or urinary tract onto the abdomen to collect waste (either faeces or urine). Stomas to collect faeces connect to the intestine and are usually formed to take pressure off an area further down the bowel or to collect faeces if the lower

bowel has been removed. Stomas to collect urine connect to the ureter (the tube that carries urine from the kidneys to the bladder). The section on the urinary system has more information about urostomies. The waste products are collected in a bag which sticks onto the abdomen.

A stoma is a bud-like structure that is formed when the surgeon stitches the opening of the bowel or ureter to the skin on the abdomen. Any operation that creates a stoma ends with 'ostomy'. For example, a colostomy involves the large bowel (colon), an ileostomy involves the small bowel (ileum) and a urostomy involves the urinary tract. Stomas can either be temporary or permanent.

Problems that might occur with the stomas include pain, bleeding, restricted circulation which can be indicated by the stoma changing colour, constipation, diarrhoea, smells or problems with the surrounding skin.

Stoma

Stomas can also be formed for the purposes of feeding. A jejunostomy is used for feeding directly into the bowel and a gastrostomy is a stoma that allows feeding directly into the stomach.

The Skeletal and Muscular Systems

The skeletal system is made up of bones, ligaments and tendons. It gives the body shape by forming a framework under the skin and protects organs such as the heart, lungs and brain. The skeletal system works with the muscular system to help the body move at the joints. Bones are linked together at joints by tough strap-like structures called ligaments. The bones at a joint do not touch each other directly but are cushioned by cartilage and fluid. When we are born our bones are mostly made up of cartilage and only harden when we get older.

The muscular system is made up of tissues that work with the skeletal system to control body movements. A muscle is attached to a bone by fibrous cords called tendons. Some muscles, like the ones in your legs, are voluntary, meaning that you decide when to move them. Other muscles, like the ones in your digestive and cardiovascular systems, are involuntary. This means that they are controlled automatically and you often don't even know they're at work.

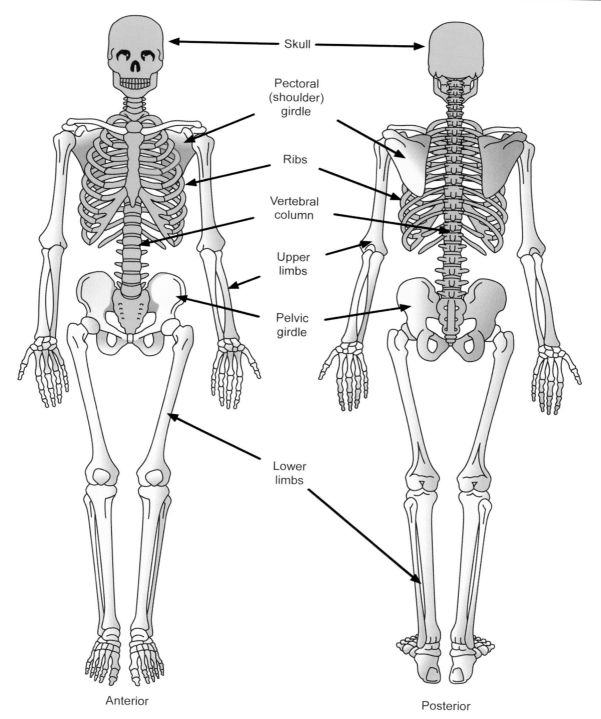

Figure 9.19 The skeletal system

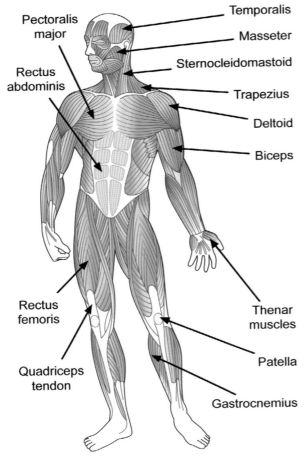

Pectoralis major

Rectus abdominis

Temporalis

Masseter

Sternocleidomastoid

Trapezius

Deltoid

Biceps

Rectus femoris

Quadriceps tendon

Thenar muscles

Patella

Gastrocnemius

Figure 9.20 The muscular system

What Can Go Wrong?

Damage to the muscles, tendons and ligaments are fairly common in both adults and children and often occur when taking part in sports and recreational activities. Injuries to muscles, tendons and ligaments vary in severity and range from simple over-stretching injuries to partial and complete tears. It is this severity that determines the level of care the person needs. Most of these types of injuries are minor and can be managed at home, but in order to able to advise people safely, we need to try and establish the severity of the injury.

It can be tricky to assess the severity of injuries affecting the muscular and skeletal systems since these bits of the body are below the skin. Occasionally, with more serious injuries, it may be possible to see the effects through the skin. For example, a broken bone may occasionally pierce the skin or there may be an obvious change in the shape of a limb indicating a fracture (broken bone) or dislocation. One of the things we can do when trying to estimate the seriousness of an injury in the absence of obvious signs is to ask the person how badly they are affected by it.

Strains

These are commonly referred to as 'pulled muscles'. These occur when a strong force suddenly pulls a muscle or tendon, causing it to tear. Poor lifting technique, or slips/trips/falls are common causes. This type of injury occurs most commonly in the legs or back, but also happens frequently in the neck.

Sprains

This is where there is an injury to a ligament. A sudden forceful twist can cause bones to come apart at the joint, resulting in a torn ligament. This is a very common sports injury. Typical sites for sprains are wrists, ankles and knees.

Dislocations

These happen when a bone actually slips out of its joint. When this type of injury occurs, there is usually very little doubt, because the joint will look very misshapen. Falls are the most common cause of dislocations. However, some people are prone to spontaneous dislocations, where very little force is needed for the bone to slip out of its joint. Most joints can be affected but the most common sites are shoulders, knees, ankles and hips.

Fractures

Let's move onto fractures or broken bones. Fractures are less common than sprains and strains. They occur mainly in adults and older children, though younger children can also suffer from broken bones. Toddler bones are less brittle than adults and also have a stronger outer covering which can provide some protection against breakages. Toddlers also have much less further to fall when they trip up.

One of the complications of fractures is that broken bones have very sharp edges, which can cause damage to other parts of the body. This can include damage to blood vessels, nerves and internal organs such as the lungs and bladder. Therefore, you may find that your CDSS has questions which help rule out any other damage to the body. For example, if someone has hurt their chest you might also see a question which asks about their breathing, because broken ribs are extremely sharp and can puncture the lining of the lung.

Treatment for a fracture involves holding the ends of the broken bone in the proper position while they heal. This is known as immobilisation which can last between two and eight weeks depending on the bone. There are different ways of immobilising bones which include:

- Plaster casts, splints or plastic braces to hold fractures in position until they have healed
- Metal plates, rods and screws
- External fixators. These devices resemble scaffolding lying outside the body. They can be made of metal or carbon fibre and have steel pins that pass into the bone directly through the skin, to hold the bones in place. It is called an external fixator as it outside the body.

The Immune and Lymphatic Systems

The immune system is the body's defence against disease. Organs, tissues and cells work together to fight off harmful substances like viruses and bacteria. The body's first line of defence against germs includes the skin, mucous membranes in the nose and throat, tears and tiny nasal hairs, bleeding, passing urine and sweating. All these things, in their different ways, block germs from entering the body or flush them away. If germs do manage to enter, then the immune system really gets to work. The hard work of the immune system is done by different types of white blood cells, which work in different ways. Some act as 'lookout' sending messages to other white blood cells when germs are detected. Others surround and destroy germs, some produce antibodies to kill them while others create substances to neutralise poisons made by the germs.

An important part of our immunity is the lymphatic system. This consists of lymph vessels, filter points called lymph nodes, and the fluid that runs through the vessels, called lymph, which is made up of excess fluid from tissues, waste products and white blood cells. The spleen is also part of this system, its function being to help filter blood and fight infection. Lymph nodes (sometimes called lymph glands) are pea-sized filters found along lymph vessels all over our body.

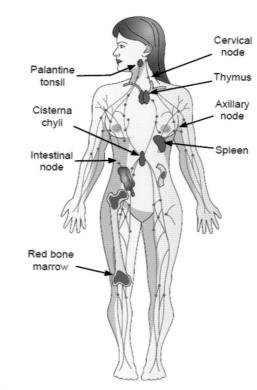

Figure 9.21 The lymphatic system

They filter and destroy toxins and germs. Lymph nodes are concentrated in the neck, armpits and groin and get bigger when fighting infection. In helping to confirm whether someone has an infection, a doctor will sometimes press on these areas to see if they are enlarged.

There are many diseases which, once you've had them, you don't catch again (for example, measles and chicken pox). So if you've already had chicken pox, your body's chicken pox antibodies make sure you don't catch it again. Vaccines work on this principle. A vaccine is a weakened form of a disease which, once inside the body, stimulates the production of antibodies. Because the disease is in a weakened form, the person who has been vaccinated will either feel very minor or no symptoms at all. The antibodies can then fight the real disease should we ever come into contact with it.

What Can Go Wrong

The immune system is constantly at work but we rarely notice it until it fails. The body's defences usually do a good job of fighting off germs, but sometimes they multiply faster than the body can handle and we become unwell. For example, every day we swallow many germs in our food and drink. Most of these die in our saliva or stomach acid, but occasionally they get through and cause food poisoning.

Another example is when we develop a cold or flu. Occasionally the germs that we constantly breathe in get past our immune system and cause an infection. Although this is a sign that the immune system has failed to eliminate the germ, the fact that we recover shows that the immune system is able to eliminate it once it has learned about it.

> ## Time out activity – signs and symptoms of wound infections
>
> Most of us have experienced or seen an infected cut, spot or sore at some point. Use this experience to think through some of the key characteristics of infected wounds

Signs of a wound infection include pain, redness and swelling which are getting worse, pus, a fever, red streaks spreading out from the wound, enlarged lymph nodes and a wound which isn't healing.

Immunocompromise

The immune system is the body's defence against infection. It is made up of a network of cells, tissues and organs that work together to protect the body. Through a series of steps called the 'immune response', the immune system attacks organisms and substances that invade body systems and cause disease, therefore reducing the chance of a serious infection developing. One of the main types of cells involved are white blood cells. A white blood cell called a 'neutrophil' is the most common infection-fighting white blood cell, and you may hear a patient say they are 'neutropenic' as a way of describing their low immunity.

When the body's immune system is weakened or not working, individuals are described as 'immunocompromised'. Another term that is sometimes used is 'immune suppressed'. This means their body is less capable of fighting organisms, which means that infections are much more likely to occur.

There are many factors that can affect the immune system, such as emotional stress, lack of sleep or poor diet, but the main conditions/factors that can seriously weaken the immune system fall into three main categories:

- Medical treatment induced immunocompromise, such as that caused by chemotherapy, radiotherapy or the drugs taken following an organ transplant.
- Conditions that a person develops/acquires at some point in their life, such as cancer, HIV/AIDS or having their spleen removed (often due to an accident of some sort).
- Conditions that a person is born with that affect the immune system.

Because infection is more likely in a person who is immunocompromised, more care is needed in managing even very minor illnesses. Included in the NHS Pathways system are questions to help you identify these people so that they can be referred quickly to their GP. Additionally, people may tell you that they have a problem with their immune system that means they must be managed in a certain way if they become ill. They may have a care plan, or firm instructions from a healthcare professional which sets out what to do in different circumstances.

The Immune System in Overdrive

Sometimes the immune system gets it wrong and tries to fight off things that aren't really a threat. Allergies are an example of this. With allergies the immune system decides to react to something that it should ignore. An allergen is the name given to a substance that can trigger an allergy such as house dust mites, pollen, foods and animal fur. Most people who've had an allergic reaction in the past know what caused it and will know if they've come into contact with the allergen again. You may get calls from people declaring that they themselves or someone else is having an allergic reaction.

Alternatively, it may be evident to you from the symptoms that a person is describing that an allergic reaction has occurred. The symptoms depend on the severity of the reaction but often include:

- Watering, itchy, red eyes
- Gritty feeling in the eyes
- Sneezing

- Itchy throat and palate
- Runny/blocked nose
- Loss of smell or taste
- Urticaria (hives – an itchy rash that looks like nettle rash)
- Digestive disturbances (in food allergies).

Anaphylaxis or anaphylactic shock is a sudden, very severe allergic reaction. It usually occurs in response to food such as peanuts. It can also be caused by other things such as venom from bee and wasp stings and drugs such as antibiotics. The initial reaction is swelling and itching in the area where the allergen entered. However, this local reaction can occur with less serious allergies. What makes anaphylaxis different is the way it quickly affects the whole body. Urticaria may develop all over the body and swelling of the face, tongue and throat make breathing difficult. Blood pressure can drop and, if left untreated, the person will collapse and lose consciousness.

Anaphylaxis must be treated urgently as the symptoms develop so quickly. A person with anaphylaxis needs emergency treatment with an injection of adrenaline. People who have previously had a serious allergic reaction often have an adrenaline injection kit with them in case of future reactions.

Further Information on Sepsis

Sepsis is the body's reaction to an infection causing the body to attack its own organs and tissues. The infection can start anywhere in the body and may either be confined to one part of the body or it may be more widespread. When someone has sepsis, their immune system triggers a series of reactions including widespread inflammation, swelling and blood clotting. This causes a significant drop in blood pressure and the blood supply to vital organs such as the brain, heart and kidneys is reduced. This is the reason someone suffering from sepsis may appear a ghastly colour and their skin may feel cold. If not recognised and treated quickly, sepsis can eventually lead to multiple organ failure and death.

Most cases of sepsis are caused by common bacteria with which we all come into contact every day without becoming ill. Sometimes, however, the body responds abnormally to these infections, causing sepsis. We do not always know why the body responds in this way; often people who get sepsis are in good health and do not have any long-term illness. However, there are some factors which increase the risk of severe sepsis:

- Being very young or very old
- Diabetes
- Taking long-term steroids or drugs to treat cancer (chemotherapy)
- Taking anti-rejection drugs after an organ transplant
- Patients with illnesses that affect the immune system (the way your body protects itself from infection), for example, leukaemia
- Having an infection or complication after an operation
- Pregnancy or very recent childbirth.

There are many similarities between the early stage of sepsis and other more common illnesses, such as flu, which can make it difficult for a healthcare professional to diagnose it in the early stages. These early symptoms include:

- Feeling cold and shivery
- Feeling hot to touch and looking flushed
- High temperature, aching muscles, tiredness
- Sickness and/or diarrhoea
- Poor appetite
- Appearing confused, drunk or having slurred speech
- Rapid breathing or difficulty breathing.

As the infection continues, it can cause a patient to feel breathless, look extremely pale/grey/blue and they may have the non-fading rash we discussed earlier. As sepsis progresses, organs become deprived of blood and oxygen, which may cause irreversible damage to the kidneys, lungs, brain and heart. Urine production reduces and breathing difficulty may increase. A person with sepsis is often confused and at risk of becoming unconscious. People with life-threatening sepsis will exhibit signs of shock.

Sepsis is a very serious illness, and sadly sometimes patients can die because they don't get treatment in time or their body is not able to fight the infection. It can be a terrible shock if a patient dies of sepsis, because the illness can move very quickly and they may have been in good health before it happened.

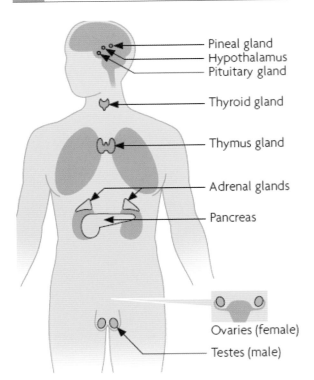

- Pineal gland
- Hypothalamus
- Pituitary gland
- Thyroid gland
- Thymus gland
- Adrenal glands
- Pancreas
- Ovaries (female)
- Testes (male)

Figure 9.22 The endocrine system

The Endocrine System

The endocrine system is made up of a group of glands that release chemical messengers or hormones into the bloodstream. This includes glands such as the pituitary, thyroid, pancreas, adrenals, ovaries and testes. Although there are many different hormones, each one affects only the cells that are programmed to respond to its message.

One of the important functions under hormonal control is the process of puberty. This generally begins sometime between the ages of 9–13 in girls and 10–15 in boys. This has implications for anyone assessing young people. Many young people are sexually active and therefore at risk of pregnancy and sexually transmitted infections at a surprisingly young age.

What Can Go Wrong?

The wrong amount of any hormone can be harmful. In some people the thyroid gland, which is situated in the neck, produces either too much or too little thyroxine, the hormone it makes. This regulates metabolism, which is the name for how the body uses and stores energy. As thyroxine levels rise, so does the speed at which chemical reactions occur in the body. Hypothyroidism, or an underactive thyroid, means you have too little thyroxine. This causes metabolism to slow down producing symptoms such as tiredness, low mood, feeling the cold, weight gain, dry skin and hair, constipation and menstrual irregularities. The opposite is hyperthyroidism, or an overactive thyroid, where the thyroid gland produces too much thyroxine. This increases the body's metabolism causing symptoms such as weight loss, increased appetite, nervousness, heat intolerance, increased bowel movements and menstrual irregularities.

Diabetes

Another disorder affecting the endocrine system in both adults and children is diabetes. This condition makes it hard for the body to control glucose levels in the blood. Under normal circumstances the hormone insulin, which is made by glands in the pancreas, carefully controls how much glucose is in the blood. Insulin helps move glucose from the bloodstream into the cells for them to use as energy. After a meal, the level of glucose in the blood rises, triggering the release of insulin. When blood glucose levels fall, for instance during exercise, insulin levels fall.

There are different types of diabetes. In Type 1 diabetes the person needs insulin injections because their pancreas makes little or no insulin. In Type 2 diabetes the pancreas does make insulin but the body is resistant to it, often because of obesity. Some patients with Type 2 diabetes need insulin, some need tablets, while others can control it with diet and exercise. Diabetes can also start in pregnancy. This is called gestational, or pregnancy-induced, diabetes. This usually goes away after the baby is born.

People with diabetes have to carefully control their blood sugar. Too much insulin or too little sugar in the blood can cause hypoglycaemia (low blood sugar), sometimes called a 'hypo'. Too little insulin or too much sugar in the blood can cause hyperglycaemia (high blood sugar). Both these conditions are harmful for the body and, in their advanced stages, are emergency situations.

Prolonged high blood sugar levels can cause the person to become drowsy before gradually drifting into unconsciousness. Other symptoms include warm, dry skin, rapid breathing, fruity

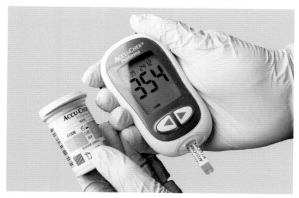

Figure 9.23 Blood glucose meter

smelling breath (often likened to pear drop sweets) and thirst. Low blood sugar affects brain function; unlike with high blood sugar, the person can become unconscious very quickly. Other symptoms include weakness, hunger, behaviour change (for example aggression or seeming to be drunk) and cold, clammy skin.

Some people with diabetes may carry their own blood testing kits and are often well prepared for emergencies (for example some diabetics keep a glucose gel with them in case of a hypo). Alternatively, they may carry a sugary drink or food. These are only suitable to use if the person is conscious and able to swallow. Some diabetics carry a glucagon injection kit in case of a severe hypoglycaemic attack. This is hormone that opposes the action of insulin. It can be administered to an unconscious person.

Diabetes also makes people prone to long-term complications such as heart disease, stroke, eye problems, kidney problems and nerve damage. People with poorly controlled diabetes are more at risk of infections (such as chest, skin and urine infections).

Adrenal Insufficiency (Addison's Disease)

Adrenal insufficiency is caused by a lack of the steroid hormones, cortisol and aldosterone, produced by the adrenal glands. Cortisol is responsible for mobilising nutrients, modifying the body's response to inflammation, stimulating the liver to raise blood sugar and helping to regulate fluid levels in the body. Aldosterone regulates salt and water levels which affects blood volume and blood pressure.

Once diagnosed, the condition can be controlled with medication. However, during times of intense stress such as during an illness, following an accident or surgery, the body needs more aldosterone and cortisol. Failure to meet these needs can lead to an adrenal crisis. This is a potentially life-threatening drop in blood pressure which can lead to unconsciousness unless the person receives hydrocortisone. People diagnosed with the disease should carry a hydrocortisone injection kit.

The Urinary System

The urinary system eliminates waste from the body, in the form of urine. After your body has taken what it needs from food, waste products are left behind in both the blood and the bowel. The bowel mainly clears the solid waste while the kidneys remove unwanted salts and chemical waste from the blood. The waste combines with water to form urine.

The kidneys are located in the fleshy part of the back between the bottom of the rib cage and the top of the hips on either side in an area called the flank. The kidneys remove waste from the blood through tiny filters. It then travels down two tubes called ureters to the bladder. Muscles in the ureter walls push urine downwards away from the kidneys. If urine is allowed to stand still, or back up, a kidney infection can develop. Small amounts of urine are emptied into the bladder from the ureters about every 10 to 15 seconds so the bladder is never completely empty.

The bladder is a hollow muscular organ that inflates when it is full and gets smaller when empty. It sits in the pelvis and stores urine until we are ready to pass it. Muscles called sphincters help stop urine leaking out. In most people the sphincter muscles close tightly like a rubber band around the opening of the bladder into the urethra, the tube that allows urine to pass outside the body.

Nerves in the bladder tell you when it is time to empty it. When you urinate, the brain signals the bladder muscles to tighten, squeezing urine out. At the same time, the brain tells the sphincters to relax. As the muscles relax, urine exits the bladder through the urethra. When all signals occur in the correct order, normal urination occurs.

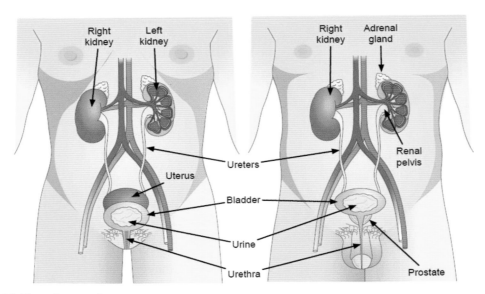

Figure 9.24 The urinary system

What Can Go Wrong?

Problems with the urinary system can be caused by injury, illness or the ageing process. As we get older, changes in the structure of the kidneys cause them to lose some of their ability to filter waste from the blood. Also, muscles in the ureters, bladder and urethra tend to lose some of their strength. Urine infections may increase because the bladder muscles do not tighten enough to empty the bladder completely. A decrease in strength of muscles of the sphincters and the pelvis can also cause incontinence – the unwanted leakage of urine.

People of any age can suffer from infections of the urinary system. Urinary tract infections are caused by bacteria in the urine that can affect either the bladder or one or both kidneys.

Infections of the kidney can cause serious damage if left untreated. These infections are usually caused by germs from the person's own bowel. These are harmless in the bowel but can cause infection if they get into other parts of the body. Women are more prone to urine infections because their urethra is shorter and opens nearer the back passage. Pregnant women are especially prone to urine infections due to hormone changes affecting the urinary tract. Urine infections in pregnant women can bring on early labour, which is one of the reasons for testing urine during pregnancy.

Time out activity – signs and symptoms of urinary tract infections

Urinary tract infections are quite common and most people have come across someone who has had one. Before reading on, try and think of three or four symptoms caused by urinary tract infections.

The main symptoms of a urinary tract infection are:
- Stinging or burning when passing urine
- Passing urine more often
- Needing to hurry to the toilet
- Blood in the urine
- Cloudy or smelly urine
- Abdominal and/or flank pain
- Fever
- Feeling unwell.

Another problem you may come across is people have difficulty passing urine. They may only be able to pass small dribbles or none at all. This condition, known as urinary retention, affects mainly older people and has different causes. Common causes include an obstruction in the urinary system or a problem affecting the nerves controlling the bladder. This is extremely uncomfortable and needs prompt treatment.

You may occasionally receive calls from people who are experiencing problems with a urinary catheter. This is a plastic tube that drains urine continuously from the bladder into a collection bag. Some catheters are inserted into the bladder via the urethra; a urethral catheter, whereas some are inserted straight into the bladder via an incision (cut) in the lower abdomen; a suprapubic catheter. Both types of catheters can become blocked and having one also increases the risk of urine infections.

Callers may also contact your service about urinary stomas or 'urostomies'. A urostomy is a permanent stoma formed if the bladder has had to be removed, or is diseased or damaged in some way. Urine drains from the stoma and collects in a pouch which is worn on the abdomen.

Injuries Affecting the Urinary System

The urinary system can become damaged when a person suffers an injury. The kidneys can be damaged by sharp or heavy blows to the flank. Less commonly, the bladder can be injured by blows in the pelvic area, but generally the pelvis provides good protection. The urethra can also become damaged if sharp objects are pushed into it.

Another way in which the kidneys can become damaged as a result of trauma is when someone has suffered a crushing injury. As has already been mentioned, this may be due to direct force from the injury or due to a process called 'crush syndrome'. Traffic and construction site accidents are the most common cause of such injuries, which can cause fractures, internal bleeding, soft tissue and organ damage. There is also a danger associated with prolonged crushing of over 15 minutes whereby there may be extensive damage to body tissues, especially muscles. Once the pressure is relieved, shock may develop as tissue fluid leaks into injured areas. Also, toxic substances collect in damaged muscle, which if released suddenly into the circulation, can cause kidney failure. Crush syndrome can prove fatal.

The Reproductive System

The Female Reproductive System

This consists of those organs that enable a woman to produce eggs, to have sexual intercourse, to

nourish a growing baby until it is fully developed and to give birth. Unlike in males, the female sexual organs are almost entirely hidden. The female organs are made up of the vagina, the uterus, the Fallopian tubes, and the ovaries, which produce the eggs. Also part of the reproductive system are the breasts that produce milk after childbirth. Once women reach sexual maturity, they experience a monthly cycle, controlled by hormones, called the menstrual cycle. These hormones control the release of an egg from one of the ovaries each month. This causes the uterine lining to thicken so it can receive a fertilised egg. Mature eggs are released from the ovary and move along the Fallopian tube. If an egg is fertilised, it tries to embed itself in the uterine wall, ready to develop into a fetus. If no egg becomes implanted, the lining is shed as menstrual blood.

Normally, after fertilisation, the fertilised embryo implants itself in the uterus and begins to develop. Occasionally, however, the embryo may embed elsewhere along its path to the uterus and begin to grow there. This is called an ectopic pregnancy and occurs in about two out of every 100 pregnancies. Sites where ectopic pregnancy may occur include the Fallopian tubes (most ectopic pregnancies occur here), the cervix, ovary or the abdominal cavity.

There is no chance of a normal pregnancy or delivery in ectopic pregnancy. In many cases, as the ectopic embryo starts to grow, it bursts the organ (usually the Fallopian tube) that contains it,

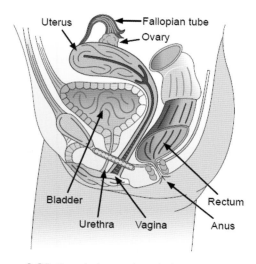

Figure 9.25 Female internal genitalia

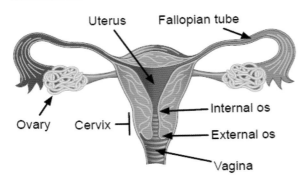

Figure 9.26 The uterus

which is said to have 'ruptured'. This can cause bleeding, severe pain, and can be life-threatening. If a woman has an ectopic pregnancy, she may experience typical early pregnancy symptoms, such as nausea and breast tenderness. Or, she may have no symptoms at all and may not even realise that she is pregnant. About a week after the first missed menstrual period, she may notice:

- Slight vaginal bleeding, which is often mistaken for a period.
- Lower abdominal pain, felt mainly on one side.

Fortunately, tests can identify an ectopic pregnancy early, before it becomes dangerous. Without treatment, the symptoms of the ectopic pregnancy will progress over several days or weeks. They include:

- Severe pelvic pain and/or lower back pain.
- Shoulder tip pain caused by blood from a ruptured ectopic pregnancy pressing on the diaphragm, the large muscle that separates the abdominal and chest cavities.
- Low blood pressure and faintness/dizziness caused by blood loss.
- Nausea and vomiting.
- Low blood pressure.

Labour and Childbirth

You may also receive calls from women in various stages of labour. Childbirth is a natural process and usually there is plenty of time to get to hospital or have a midwife present for home delivery before the baby is born. However, occasionally things don't go to plan. There are three stages of labour and it is important to understand these stages to be able to deal with calls regarding labour and childbirth.

First Stage of Labour

During this stage, the mucus plug that was in place to protect the uterus from infection is expelled. This is commonly called 'a show' and looks like blood-stained slimy mucus. Muscular contractions spread through the uterus with increasing frequency. Contractions may be felt in the back, abdomen or pelvis. Although the contractions can be very painful, there should be relatively pain-free periods between them. Severe, continuous pain can indicate that something worrying is happening to the mother or the baby. As labour progresses the contractions become more frequent and these, along with the pressure of the baby's head, cause the cervix to stretch and open up. This process can take some hours. At some point during this stage, the sac of fluid that encloses the baby (the amniotic fluid) usually bursts. As the waters break, the gush of fluid is usually clear and watery. Sometimes it also contains streaks of blood or white bits. If the fluid is green or brown-stained it may mean that the baby is getting tired or is in trouble.

Second Stage of Labour

Once the cervix is fully dilated, the baby presses down on the pelvic muscles. This causes a feeling of pressure or fullness on the back passage or vagina and an urge to push, which may feel like the need to empty the bowels. However, the mother should not be allowed to sit on the toilet. This is a sign that labour is well advanced and that the birth is likely to happen soon. The vagina stretches as the baby is pushed out and the baby will become visible at the vaginal opening. The umbilical cord looks like a thin rope made of gristle. The surface is white and shiny and the inside may look dark red or blue. Occasionally during this stage the umbilical cord may be seen hanging out of the vagina. This is known as a cord prolapse; whilst very rare, it is also very dangerous for the unborn baby.

Most babies are born head first and the top of the head is visible just before delivery. Sometimes the baby presents bottom first (breech) and labour is then usually longer and more prone to complications. Rarely a foot or shoulder may come first which makes labour very difficult. The second stage is over once the baby is born.

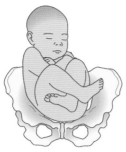

Figure 9.27 Breech birth

Third Stage of Labour

During this stage the afterbirth (placenta) is delivered. It is usually passed out of the mother's vagina between 10 and 30 minutes after the baby is born. The mother often feels some mild contractions at the time and she may feel the urge to push. When the afterbirth is delivered there is usually a gush of blood. This is normal and should settle in a few minutes. Some continued blood loss is also normal, but it should not be heavy. Severe bleeding after delivery can occur if the uterus fails to contact properly after the placenta pulls away from the uterus. This is an emergency situation.

The Male Reproductive System

The male reproductive system enables a man to have sexual intercourse and to fertilise the ovum with sperm. The sexual organs of the male are

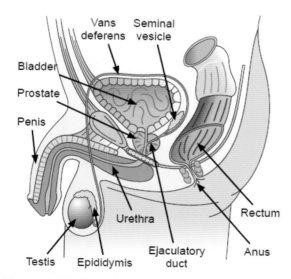

Figure 9.28 The male reproductive system

partly visible and partly hidden within the body. The visible parts are the penis and the scrotum. Sperm and male sex hormones are produced in the testes, a pair of oval-shaped glands. These are suspended in the scrotum, which hangs outside the body cavity. This ensures that sperm are kept below the body temperature, which is essential for healthy sperm production. Inside the body are glands called the prostate gland and seminal vesicles; these provide lubricating fluids that nourish the sperm. Inside the body sperm passes out of the testes through a long tube comprising the epididymis and vas deferens. Sperm leaves the body through the tube that also carries urine, the urethra.

What Can Go Wrong?

In men there is a condition where a testicle can become twisted within the scrotum, cutting off the blood supply. This leads to sudden pain and swelling in the testicular area. It is very serious and needs prompt treatment to save the testicle and the future ability to have children.

Lumps and swelling can affect the ovaries in women and the testicles in men. As with lumps everywhere they need checking to exclude anything serious. In the testicle in particular, just because a lump isn't painful doesn't mean it can be ignored. Early detection of testicular cancer makes a huge difference to survival rates.

Women often do not know they have ovarian swelling until they develop a pain. Some ovarian swellings are filled with fluid (ovarian cysts). If they burst the woman will often feel sudden severe pain in her lower abdomen and needs urgent attention.

In pregnant women, a common occurrence is miscarriage. This is the loss of an unborn baby before the twenty-fourth week of pregnancy. Symptoms can include vaginal bleeding ranging from light spotting to heavy blood loss, abdominal cramps, pain in the pelvic area and backache. Some minor vaginal bleeding is common during pregnancy and bleeding does not always signal a miscarriage, especially if it is light and only lasts a short time. Following a miscarriage or a termination, dead tissue may remain in the womb and increase the risk of infection and vaginal discharge.

Sexually transmitted infections (STIs) can occur in both men and women. If left untreated, they may cause permanent damage, such as infertility and even death.

The symptoms of a sexually transmitted infection include:

- An unusual genital discharge
- Itching, soreness or inflammation in the genital area
- Pain passing urine
- Bleeding between periods
- Pain during sex
- Abdominal pain
- Testicular pain/swelling
- Sores, rashes and warts on the genitals and other parts of the body
- Feeling unwell.

STIs can be diagnosed and treated at genitourinary medicine (GUM) clinics. The person can attend without giving their name if they wish to and their GP won't be informed without their consent. People can be very embarrassed when discussing problems associated with the reproductive system, and great sensitivity is required from everyone involved.

It is important to remember that when someone has an STI they may have one, several or none of these symptoms. Also many of these symptoms occur with disorders other than STIs. As we know, our role is never to diagnose. What we must do, however, is pick up symptoms that need further assessment whatever the cause.

The Senses

There are five senses: sight, hearing, touch, smell and taste. Here we consider each sense and the parts of the body responsible, but we will pay most attention to the eyes and skin as these often generate quite a lot of calls to telephone triage services.

Sight – The Eyes

These complex structures allow us to see what is going on around us. The eyeball has a tough, white outer covering called the sclera. The part of the sclera in front of the coloured part of the eye is called the cornea. This part is transparent to let light through. Behind the cornea is the coloured part of the eye, the iris. This controls the amount of light getting into the eye through the pupil, the black circle in the centre of the eye. Once through

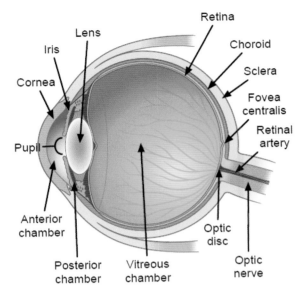

Figure 9.29 Eye structures

the pupil, light hits the lens. This clear structure projects light onto the retina at the back of the eye. The retina contains cells which are sensitive to light. These cells generate nerve signals that are carried to the brain via the optic nerve. The bulk of the eyeball is filled with a clear jelly called the vitreous humour. The front of the eye is protected by the eyelid and each blink bathes the eye with tears. This helps wash away germs or other particles that could harm the eye.

What Can Go Wrong?

Various problems can occur with the eyes. Injuries are quite common, ranging from small scratches and foreign bodies in the eye to serious accidents which can cause blindness. Scratches can be caused by fingernails, make-up brushes and pencils, contact lenses, twigs and dust. Often this causes watering, redness of the eye and a gritty sensation. If the symptoms persist it is important that the eye is examined in case the cornea is damaged. More serious eye injuries can be caused by chemical splashes that can burn the eye. Bleaches, strong acids and alkalis are very painful and can cause a lot of damage to the eye. The cornea can also be damaged by exposure to ultraviolet light, such as the glare from sunlight reflected off snow or a welder's torch.

Minor eye infections are common in adults and children. The main symptom is a thick, discoloured discharge from one or both eyes. With minor infections the person still feels well. However, serious infections of the eye socket do very occasionally occur. This causes a painful swelling of an eyelid, which can be so swollen it is impossible to open the eye. This occurs in both adults and children and needs urgent treatment. With this serious eye infection the person will feel very ill.

Hearing – The Ears

As well as allowing us to hear, the ears also help us to balance. Sound waves are funnelled into the outer ear; the bit we can see on the outside. Sound travels down the ear canal, causing the eardrum at the end to vibrate. The eardrum touches three tiny bones that are linked together and the vibrations pass along these bones. The last of the three bones touches a fluid-filled structure shaped like a snail's shell called the cochlea. The vibrations move the fluid inside the cochlea which stimulates nerves to carry the signal to the brain. These signals are interpreted as sounds. As well as providing our sense of hearing, part of the ear's job is also to give our brains information that helps us to keep our balance and coordinate our movements.

What Can Go Wrong?

It is not uncommon for a foreign body to become lodged in the ear. This can cause temporary deafness and in some cases, damage to the eardrum. A perforated ear drum can also be caused by a blow to the side of the head, an explosion or a significant change in atmospheric pressure. Earache is a very common condition especially in children. The most common cause is infection, which can either be viral or bacterial. Many cases of earache clear up without treatment and don't require antibiotics. Some ear problems can upset a person's balance, causing them to become extremely dizzy. Because the brain is affected by not getting the right information from the balance mechanism in the ear, the person may vomit or feel sick, or may fall and be unable to get up again.

Touch – The Skin

The skin is a very important organ and carries out several vital functions. The outer layer of skin is the epidermis. The inner layer is called the dermis. This contains hair follicles, nerves, sweat and oil glands and blood vessels. It acts as a protective layer over the body and helps prevent injury and disease. It also maintains moisture in the body, getting rid of waste and regulating body temperature via our sweat glands and skin circulation. A network of nerve endings all over the body sends messages to the brain about pressure and temperature on the skin.

What Can Go Wrong?

Many things can damage the skin since this part of the body is in constant contact with the outside world. Damage ranges from very minor cuts and grazes to large wounds or burns. There are several different types of wounds:

- *Abrasions* (grazes) occur when the top layer of skin is scraped off. Rope burns, carpet burns, and skinned knees or elbows are common examples. This kind of wound can become infected quite easily because dirt and germs are usually embedded in the tissues.

- *Incisions* are wounds made by sharp cutting instruments such as knives, razors, and broken glass. Incisions tend to bleed freely because the blood vessels are cut cleanly. Structures such as tendons, nerves and arteries may become damaged. Incisions are less likely to become infected, as the blood flow often flushes out harmful germs.

- *Lacerations* are tears, rather than cuts. They have ragged, irregular edges and may have torn tissue underneath. Unlike incisions these

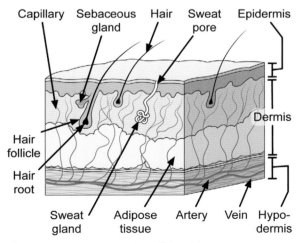

Figure 9.30 Cross-section of the skin

wounds are caused by more blunt objects. A wound made by a blunt knife, for instance, is more likely to be a laceration than an incision. Bomb fragments often cause lacerations. Many of the wounds caused by accidents with machinery are lacerations. Lacerations are frequently contaminated with dirt, grease or other material that is ground into the tissue. They are therefore prone to infection.

- *Punctures* are caused by objects that penetrate into the tissues leaving only a small surface opening. Wounds made by nails, needles, wire and bullets are usually punctures. As a rule, small puncture wounds may cause severe internal bleeding. The possibility of infection is great in all puncture wounds, as bacteria is often pushed deep into the wound.
- *Amputation* is the severing of a body part such as a leg or arm. Bleeding is often heavy and shock may develop. The body part can often be successfully reattached.

Time out activity – burns

Another problem you are likely to receive calls about is burns. Nearly everyone has had a burn at some time or another. Spend a couple of minutes thinking about how a burn looks and feels before reading on.

The cause of a burn may be direct heat such as flames and hot surfaces, electrical, or chemical.

A burn caused by a hot fluid is called a scald. The damage caused by burns varies enormously depending on factors such as what caused the burn, its location, the size of the person, how quickly the burn was treated and so on.

When skin is damaged it functions less effectively as a barrier against germs, and infections can occur. Additionally, body fluids may be lost due to fluid leaking into blisters or through the skin surface. If fluid loss is very large, the circulation can become depleted and shock can develop, which is life-threatening. Burns are classified according to how deep they are, and can be superficial, partial thickness or full thickness. These are explained further in Figure 9.31 below.

Minor burns can be treated at home, but deep or large burns need to be carefully assessed and treated in hospital. Burns on certain parts of the body, such as the face, hands, feet, or around large joints and genitals, also require further assessment since they are more prone to complications.

Smell and Taste – The Nose and Tongue

The nasal cavities and the mouth form the entrance to the respiratory system. The nasal cavities are lined with small hairs and cells that produce mucus to trap debris. Within the nasal cavities is an area with millions of smell-sensitive

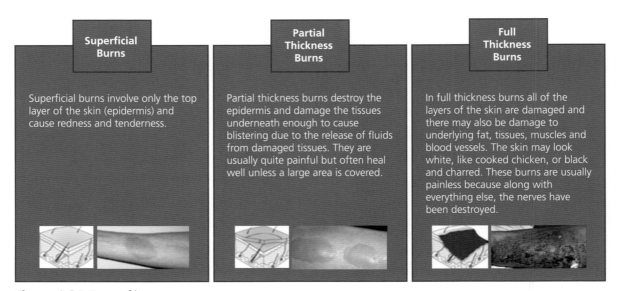

Figure 9.31 Types of burns

Source: NHS Pathways Distance Learning Pack, NHS Digital

cells. These have tiny hairs onto which odour particles stick. This produces nerve signals that travel to the brain to be interpreted as smells. Your sense of smell warns you of dangers such as smoke and poisonous gases.

The tongue is covered in taste buds. Different parts of the tongue are sensitive to different flavours: sweet, salt, sour and bitter. This protects the body from ingesting unsafe substances. Foods that are poisonous or rotten usually taste bad which means that we are less likely to eat them. In order to taste things fully we also require the sense of smell.

What Can Go Wrong?

Young children often push small objects into the nose, which can block it and cause infection or damage. It is important that parents/carers should not try to remove the object, since this often pushes it further into the nose.

As well as the obvious cold symptoms we are all familiar with, another common complaint associated with the nose is sinusitis. The sinuses are air-filled cavities in the skull behind the bones of the face and forehead that open up into the nasal cavity. Air passes through these spaces, and mucus drains through them and out of the nose. Anything that causes the lining of the nasal passages to swell, such as allergy or infection, can block the opening to the sinuses and lead to sinusitis. Symptoms include facial pain and headache (especially when leaning forwards), nasal obstruction often with thick yellow/green discharge, fever, bad breath, diminished sense of smell, fatigue, tooth pain and sometimes cough.

A common condition affecting the tongue and inside of the mouth is mouth ulcers. Usually about 3–5mm in diameter, they are most commonly caused by trauma to the mouth such as biting the tongue or cheek, but are also thought to be caused by an overreaction by the body's own immune system. Mouth ulcers usually get better on their own but ulcers which persist for longer than three weeks should be assessed by a healthcare professional. Repeated mouth ulcers can be part of several medical conditions; very rarely a mouth ulcer can be cancerous.

Summary

Having a sound understanding of some basic anatomy and physiology will support your everyday practice as a call handler and help you carry out your role sensitively and effectively. The CDSS that you are using will have been built by people who are experts in the human body and how it functions, but it's important that you understand some basic principles of anatomy and physiology too. If ever you are in doubt about something 'medical' presented to you by a caller, make sure you seek some clinical advice straightaway.

References and Further Reading

Material in this chapter has been reproduced from: Richard Pilbery and Kris Lethbridge, *Ambulance Care Practice*, Bridgwater: Class Publishing (2016), with kind permission from the authors.

Waugh, A. and Grant, A. (2018). *Ross & Wilson: Anatomy and Physiology in Health and Illness*, 13th edition. Oxford: Elsevier.

Chapter 10: Health and Wellbeing at Work

Learning Objectives

By the end of this chapter you will be able to:

- Describe a range of measures aimed at staying healthy at work such as headset hygiene or hand-washing
- Describe the main physical hazards within a call centre environment and state the importance of addressing these appropriately
- State the case for emotional wellbeing at work
- Describe the impact of work on our mental health
- Describe practical ideas for promoting effective wellbeing
- Summarise what is meant by mindfulness and how this can be a useful strategy within a call handling role
- Explain the potential impact of shift work on wellbeing and how this can be minimised.

Introduction

Employers have a duty to ensure the workplace of their staff meets health and safety standards and that processes are in place to control health and safety risks. It is their responsibility to ensure you are fully trained in your role and to provide you with the knowledge and skills to identify risks and how to report them. The employer should provide the necessary equipment required for you to carry out your job safely.

The primary responsibility for health and safety lies with the employer, however that being said, the employee also has a responsibility to ensure that they follow any health and safety guidelines. You need to take care not to put others at risk with your actions, not to misuse any equipment and always to report any identified risks that may cause harm to yourself or others.

The Physical Workplace

Headsets

Headsets can be worn for prolonged periods of time when working in a call handling environment. It is therefore important that they fit comfortably, are well maintained, are cleaned regularly and are fit for purpose. It may not always be possible, but it is strongly recommended that

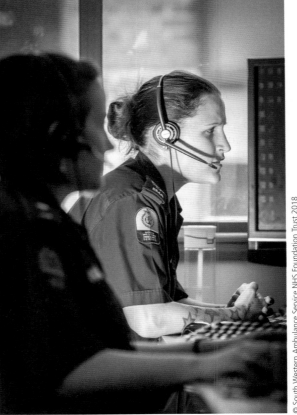

© South Western Ambulance Service NHS Foundation Trust 2018

Figure 10.1 Headsets may be worn for a prolonged period of time when working in a call handling environment

headsets should be personal issue or at least the ear pads and voice pad, to avoid risk of infection. The volume controls should be adjusted to suit each individual. If the volume is turned up to hear a quieter caller, do not forget to readjust it for the next caller.

Call handling centres can be very noisy areas to work in due to the amount of staff and number of calls coming in. Some staff may struggle to block out the background noise and distractions. There are noise-cancelling headsets that can help to minimise background noise. Some people may prefer a bilateral headset (with two ear pieces) to assist with cancelling out other sounds within the centre.

Regular hearing assessments are recommended to identify any changes in the hearing so they can be managed effectively, ensuring that each individual is allocated a headset that meets their requirements. Hearing is clearly a critical sense within this type of role. Regular eye tests are also important to detect any changes.

Work Stations

Using equipment such as visual display screens and carrying out repetitive tasks every day can lead to a number of physical problems, particularly if the equipment is not used correctly, if there is poor posture or if regular breaks are not taken.

Prolonged or incorrect use of visual display equipment can give rise to conditions such as fatigue, eye strain and musculoskeletal aches and pains. Ideally, a workplace assessment should be carried out and training given on how equipment should be placed for each individual's needs. Hot desking is commonplace, but on each shift you should adjust the workstation to suit your own requirements. A workplace assessment may consider the following factors:

- Display screens and keyboard requirements
- Desk height
- Foot and wrist supports
- Mouse requirements
- Chair and work posture
- Layout
- Lighting, heating and ventilation
- Noise.

According to the Chartered Institute of Ergonomics and Human Factors (2016), research has shown

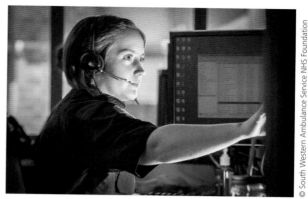

Figure 10.2 On each shift you should adjust the workplace to suit your own requirements

that effective office ergonomics interventions on average reduce the number of musculoskeletal problems by 61%, reduce lost workdays by 88% and reduce staff turnover by 87%.

Hygiene

As previously mentioned, most call handling centres operate a hot desk policy. Taking responsibility for keeping desk areas clean is important not only for your own welfare, but also for the welfare of your colleagues.

Handwashing is widely acknowledged to be the single most effective measure for preventing the spread of infection. If you have a cold, then ensure you wash your hands regularly and dispose of any tissues appropriately. Figure 10.3 shows the technique for effective hand washing.

Wiping down your desk should be part of your preparation at the beginning of each shift. Some call handling centres may have rules in place around what you are allowed to have at your desk, in an attempt to keep them clean and avoid spillages onto electrical equipment. If you are allowed to eat and drink at your desk, be considerate of any colleagues with serious food allergies.

These rules are in place to help break the chain of infection shown in Figure 10.4 that starts with an **INFECTIOUS AGENT**. This is a microbial organism with the ability to cause disease. The greater the organism's ability to grow and multiply, enter tissue and cause disease, the greater the possibility that the organism will cause an infection. Infectious agents are bacteria, viruses, fungi, and parasites.

WASH HANDS WHEN VISIBLY SOILED! OTHERWISE, USE HANDRUB

Duration of the entire procedure: 40–60 seconds

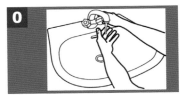

Wet hands with water;

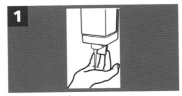

Apply enough soap to cover all hand surfaces;

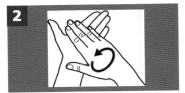

Rub hands palm to palm;

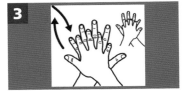

Right plam over left dorsum with interlaced fingers and vice versa;

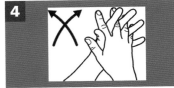

Palm to palm with fingers interlaced;

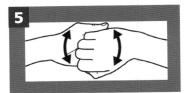

Backs of fingers to opposing palms with fingers interlocked;

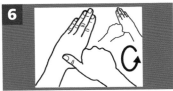

Rotational rubbing of left thumb clasped in right palm and vice versa;

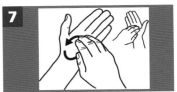

Rotational rubbing, backwards and forwards with clasped fingers of right hand in left palm and vice versa;

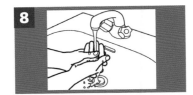

Rinse hands with water;

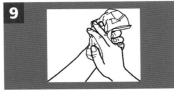

Dry hands thoroughly with a single use towel;

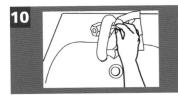

Use towel to turn off faucet;

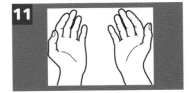

Your hands are now safe.

Figure 10.3 Handwashing technique
Source: World Health Organization (2009)

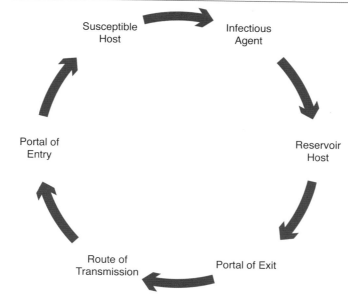

Figure 10.4 Chain of infection

The infectious agent needs a **RESERVOIR** which is a place within which microorganisms can thrive and reproduce. This may include your nose, throat and lungs. The infectious agent then needs a **PORTAL OF EXIT** which provides a way for a microorganism to leave the reservoir, for example when someone sneezes or coughs. Then there needs to be a **ROUTE OF TRANSMISSION** which is the way the organism moves or is carried from one place to another. In a call centre environment it is very likely that this may include:

- Direct contact by touch. This could be by shaking hands
- Indirect contact via contaminated equipment such as the use of shared computer keyboards
- Airborne particles from coughing and sneezing
- Faecal-oral route via poor hand hygiene.

The infectious agent then requires a **PORTAL OF ENTRY**. This includes body orifices, mucus membranes, or breaks in the skin. Thinking about your role in a call centre should enable you to identify that using a shared keyboard has the potential to provide a portal of entry, especially if you scratch your nose or put your fingers to your mouth. The infectious agent then requires a **SUSCEPTIBLE HOST**. This is someone who is susceptible to the disease or lacking immunity to overcome the infectious agent.

Hazards

There are many objects within the working environment that can cause a hazard. Common hazards within call handling centres are bags, coats or belongings left lying under desks or on the floor. This is a trip hazard and can prevent colleagues from having sufficient space to work.

What else can we look out for to make it safe for all at work?

- Loose or trailing wires/cables/headsets
- Trip hazards
- Spillages
- Electrical hazards
- Blockages to fire exits
- Hazards that could start a fire such as an overloaded plug socket.

Reporting

If you see a potential hazard then it is your responsibility to take action to prevent harm. If it is something as simple as moving a trip hazard, then do it straight away. If it is something that you cannot correct at the time or could potentially put you in danger, then report it through the appropriate route. Assess the likelihood of the hazard causing harm. This should help you determine how quickly action needs to be taken.

It is **everyone's** responsibility to prevent and/or report anything that can cause harm.

Emotional Wellbeing at Work

Your wellbeing at work matters. The Chartered Institute of Personnel and Development (2016) have this to say on the matter:

> 'Wellbeing is more than an avoidance of becoming physically sick. It represents a broader bio-psycho-social construct that includes physical, mental and social health. Well employees are physically and mentally able, willing to contribute in the workplace and likely to be more engaged at work.'

They go on to say:

> 'The wellbeing approach also brings benefits for people at all levels inside and outside the workplace. It makes the workplace a more productive, attractive and corporately responsible place to work. Positive wellbeing can also benefit the local community and, more broadly, the country as a whole because of well people requiring less support from the health services.'

So you can see that your wellbeing really matters on many different levels. There's a wealth of evidence showing that people who feel happy and healthy at work stay longer, have fewer absences and do a better job. More than that, healthy workplaces make healthy communities that use fewer precious health resources. Most importantly though, is the fact that most people spend a significant proportion of their adult lives in work, so it makes sense that this should be a time which is emotionally satisfying and happy.

The role carried out by call handlers is complex, demanding and can be emotionally draining. What you do really matters – the stakes are high, because you are often the gateway to someone getting the treatment they need. A mistake within this setting can be catastrophic, but fortunately 999 and 111 do have a very good safety record. Nonetheless, it can be a stressful and challenging role. Call handlers talk of situations such as talking a parent through how to administer CPR to a child that has stopped breathing, with tears rolling down their own face. Other call handlers talk of the joy of talking a woman through the process of labour and the 'magic' of hearing a baby's first cry.

This is obviously a happy situation to be part of, but nevertheless the strength of emotion and the adrenaline rush involved is likely to be enormous. Calls regarding mental health issues can be really challenging, particularly if a person is reporting suicidal feelings. Other call handlers talk about the abuse they receive over the telephone, and the necessity of reacting in a calm, helpful manner, particularly if someone is in need of urgent help.

The 999 and 111 services are extremely busy and demand is rising year on year. Call handlers are expected to work efficiently and in a focused way, because there is often another call waiting and who knows how urgent that might be? Services tend to be busiest outside of normal working hours, perhaps when most of your family and friends are enjoying some downtime. All of these demands, added to the public scrutiny that 999 and 111 experience, make the role extremely challenging and it can have an impact on your emotional wellbeing and mental health.

According to the mental health charity Mind, at least one in six workers experiences common mental health problems, including anxiety and depression. Their research shows that work is the biggest cause of stress in people's lives, more so than debt or other financial problems [Mind, 2013]. A 2012 US study highlights how people involved in answering emergency calls can go on to develop post-traumatic stress disorder following traumatic calls. Within the study, calls related to the death or serious injury of a child were rated as the most traumatic, closely followed by those from suicidal callers and the unexpected death of an adult. The research indicates that many call takers report symptoms of severe stress, with a small proportion reporting symptoms serious enough to be diagnosed with post-traumatic stress disorder (Pierce and Lilly, 2012).

But it is not all bad news. Many people find that being in work is good for their mental health. As well as providing an income, work can give a sense of identity and opportunities to make a difference or a contribution to the world around you. It can also provide the opportunity to connect with others, as well as providing a predictable structure and a regular routine. Whilst work can be stressful, there is a lot you can do to protect yourself from emotional burn out. There are also actions that we can take to help reduce the stigma associated with mental health. Making mental health safe and easy to talk about is important, because it helps people acknowledge when they are struggling. Seeking help, support and sometimes treatment for mental health problems is just as important as seeking help for physical ailments. However, because of the taboo associated with mental health, people find it difficult to admit they are struggling.

Some Practical Ideas to Help You Be Emotionally Well at Work

Managing your Workload and Getting the Work–Life Balance Right

- Be strict about taking your breaks. It is really important to take some time to refuel and refocus. Occasionally you may need to work longer than your set hours, but do try to get your time back at some point, otherwise you can end up feeling depleted and undervalued.

- Make sure you take regular holidays from work, throughout the year.

- Do not let work take over your whole life. Nurture and protect your outside interests and home life. You do important work, but it should only form part of your life. Take time to prioritise what's important outside of work.

- Try to create clear boundaries between work and home. Perhaps use the journey on the way home to process what's happened or wind down. Some people find that having a 'leaving work' routine can help them mark the separation between work and home.

- Learn to say 'no' when appropriate. For example, accepting overtime shifts when you are already feeling tired, stressed or overwhelmed is likely to be highly detrimental to your health and wellbeing. Make your wellbeing a priority.

Manage Stress Positively and Proactively

- Recognising what causes you to feel stressed is an important first step. Being aware of what you find difficult enables you to put appropriate preventative measures in place or to respond quickly to the first signs that things are getting too much.

- Talk to your manager about what you find difficult at work. It may be that they can support you in some way (for instance by providing some additional training about certain types of calls).

- Start talking about mental health in a general sense – get the conversation going. You do not have to reveal deeply personal things about yourself, but often you will find that if you have struggled with something, so has someone else. We all have a part to play in making mental health safer and easier to talk about at work.

- Make use of the resources available. For example, some organisations provide 'sharing groups' that enable call handlers to get together to talk about their work, particularly the more difficult aspects. If this sort of thing does not exist, how about suggesting it? All organisations should provide access to an occupational health department; some will provide access to employee assistance programmes and counselling.

- Avoid unhealthy coping mechanisms such as alcohol misuse, drug use or overeating. These only ever have a short-term effect on our mood and, in the longer term, often contribute to physical and mental ill health.

- Experiment with different coping mechanisms when you feel stress building up. The Stress Management Society (www.stress.org.uk/) has some great ideas.

- Make sure you get a good night's sleep. Sleep is essential for health. The subject is too big to cover here, but NHS Choices has some good information on promoting a healthy sleep pattern.

- The mental health charity Mind maintains a large website with comprehensive information you may find useful [www.mind.org.uk].

Foster Connections at Work

A fundamental human need is that of feeling close to and accepted and valued by others. But connections between people do not always happen automatically; sometimes it takes some effort. How about giving some of these ideas a try?

- Make an effort to get to know people within your organisation. Go out of your way to say hello and find out a little bit about people. Share information about yourself. Ask how someone's weekend was and listen properly to their reply. Look for common ground and shared interests and use this to keep connections going.

- Notice people's body language and take time to ask how they are, particularly if they seem to be struggling.
- Organise out-of-work get-togethers and activities.
- Avoid being a part of 'office gossip'. People often use this as a way of building connections with others, but it can be hurtful and very damaging.
- Give someone a lift to work or suggest sharing the journey with them.
- Don't over-rely on email as a form of communication.

Be Active

Physical activity is known to have a protective effect against common mental health issues such as anxiety and depression. It can be more difficult to incorporate activity into call centre work, but it is not impossible. Here are a few ideas:

- Walk into work or perhaps just get off the bus a stop earlier. Perhaps you could do this with a colleague.
- Go for a quick walk at lunchtime.
- Take the stairs whenever possible.
- Form a team to focus on a physical/sporting activity. Local sponsored walks or runs are a great way to keep active. Participating as part of a team can really help you bond and get to know each other.
- Do some gentle stretching before work, or in between calls at your desk. Ask your employer about the availability of stand-up desks.

Focus on Being of Service to Others

- Participation in social and community life has attracted a lot of attention in the field of wellbeing research. Individuals who report a greater interest in helping others are more likely to rate themselves as happy. Your job is completely dedicated to being of service, but have you really stopped to think about how what you do helps others? Take some time each day to think about the difference you have made today to your callers' lives. How have you helped

them? How have you reassured them? How did you demonstrate care and kindness to them?

- Try carrying out regular acts of kindness every week and see what the results are. According to Lyubomirsky and Layous (2013), people who engage in kind acts become happier over time. Lyubomirsky, who has studied happiness for over 20 years, has found that performing kind acts once a week led to increased happiness.

Engage with Lifelong Learning

- The job of a call handler is complex, demanding and ever-changing. It can feel really stressful if there are aspects of your role that you feel unprepared for. Be proactive in identifying aspects of your role that you find challenging and discuss these with your manager or training/coaching staff.
- Make it your priority to continually identify areas where you could build up your knowledge, experience and expertise, perhaps learning from more experienced colleagues or those with particular areas of expertise.
- Engage in activities like self and peer audit as a way of continually developing your practice.
- Make the most of learning opportunities and resources around you. Make it your business to find out what training resources can be assessed within your organisation.

Mindfulness at Work

You may have heard of mindfulness or perhaps even started to investigate it within your own life. It's a practice and way of approaching the world that has a great deal to offer you in your role as a call handler. At its simplest, mindfulness is about focusing on the present moment, rather than thinking about the past or the future. It takes practice to cultivate the skills of mindfulness, but it can be invaluable in helping you cope with the demands of everyday life and a stressful job.

One study showed a significant reduction in work-related worrying and chronic fatigue coupled with improvements in sleep quality, for workers who completed an online mindfulness course [Querstret et al. 2016]. There are different ways to learn about mindfulness and how to incorporate it into your daily life. There are courses (both online and traditional), books, apps, podcasts and videos. The 'Be Mindful' website is a good place to start (see www.bemindful.co.uk/). Here are some tips for you to try:

• *Mindful Breathing*. This exercise only takes one minute and could be done before work, between calls, during a break (even a toilet break!), when you're feeling stressed, anxious or upset or at the end of a shift. Nobody has to know what you're doing. All you have to do is be still and focus on your breath for just one minute.

Start by breathing in and out slowly. One in and out cycle should last for about 6–8 seconds. It doesn't matter if you breathe through your nose or mouth. See if you can focus your attention on just feeling your breath. Maybe it feels cold on the way in and warm on the way out. Maybe you can feel your chest or belly moving when you breathe. Try and let go of thoughts for this minute by focusing on your breath. If thoughts do pop up, don't worry, that often happens. Just refocus on your breathing. After the minute has passed, continue to breathe as normal, but perhaps you might try this exercise several times a day.

• *Mindful Awareness*. This practice is intended to encourage a greater appreciation of simple, everyday tasks. The effect is often that we derive greater satisfaction from doing them, as well as completing them more effectively. Choose a work-based activity that happens many times every day; something you take for granted.

Once you've chosen your activity, make a commitment for one day to focus on it intently every time you carry it out. Before you embark on the activity, take a deep breath and bring yourself completely into the present moment. This means focusing on nothing else, apart from what is happening right now. Start the activity and focus on it with all your senses (for example, it might be the process of taking down a caller's demographics or the steps you go through in explaining the call process to each caller). Avoid thinking about the last time you carried it out or the next time you'll do it; instead savour each second of doing it in the present moment. Each time you feel your attention or thoughts wandering, make a deliberate effort to refocus on the activity in question.

At the end of the day, you might choose to look back to see what the results of this practice were. Did you notice anything different? How did it feel to focus closely on this everyday activity? Were there any surprises?

• *Mindful Listening*. This is something we should all be engaging in when we're involved in telephone triage, but it can be hard work and takes practice. When you are taking a call, use the process outlined in the section above on 'mindful awareness' to focus all of your attention on what you hear over the telephone. Every time you feel your thoughts wandering or start getting caught up in distraction, make a concerted effort to refocus your attention on the sounds coming to you over the telephone. Listen to what's being said, what's being intimated and all the background noises you can hear from the caller's end. Try not to make assumptions about what you hear, and make sure you ask questions to check what you're hearing.

At the end of the call, reflect back with curiosity to see what the result of this focused, mindful listening was. Did the call feel different in any way? How did it feel to focus so closely on listening? Do you normally do this? Were there any surprises?

• *Mindful Appreciation*. This last practice simply involves searching out and noticing three things that you are grateful for or three things that went well. These do not have to be enormous momentous events, in fact it is better to focus on the small things that often go unnoticed in our lives. This simple and often enjoyable task has a strong basis in research – when we actively focus on the things we're grateful for, our brain becomes more attuned to focusing on the positive things in our life and as a result, we often tend to become happier.

The point is simply to give thanks and appreciation for what might be considered the insignificant things in life. Mostly you can do this internally, but it's also really worthwhile to actually express this gratitude to those around you. Similarly, some people find having gratitude partner(s) really helpful. Some people choose to discuss this over the dinner table with their loved ones, whilst others like to incorporate mindful appreciation into their bedtime routine.

It doesn't matter how bad your day has been, there are always things to be grateful for. These often little things play an important part in our existence, but can easily get overshadowed by our grasping after bigger pleasures and experiences. Examples might be a colleague bringing you a cup of tea, a heartfelt thank you from a patient, getting the kids out of the house with minimal fuss, the bus being on time, a smile from a stranger, a beautiful sunrise, food in the cupboards, heating that works or a hug when you get in from work. Taking time to express gratitude for the little triumphs, kindnesses and successes in your day increases your tendency to notice them in the moment which can bring a greater sense of contentment and satisfaction with your life, including your work life.

Case Study

Mohammed has been a call handler for just three months. This is his first job after university. He finds the work rewarding but also very stressful at times. He finds calls about mental health issues particularly difficult and can often feel signs of anxiety when handling such calls. These signs include a racing heart, dry mouth and fast breathing. These are all signs that Mohammed's 'fight or flight' response has been triggered. This is a normal reaction to highly stressful circumstances but it can cause us to behave in certain unhelpful ways. In Mohammed's case, these physical symptoms make him want to end the call as quickly as possible – this is the 'flight' part of the response; it causes us to want to escape the situation as quickly as possible.

Mohammed works for a forward-thinking, proactive organisation that has several initiatives in place to help staff deal with workplace stress. Mohammed talks to his manager about how he feels when dealing with such calls. His manager suggests reading a booklet that's been introduced, which focuses on breathing exercises to deal with anxiety.

Mohammed reads the booklet and decides to give it a try. He focuses on trying the breathing techniques between each call. It only takes a minute to carry out and he notices that he starts to feel calmer and more in control. Once he gets the hang of it, he starts to practice slow deep breathing whilst actually taking a call. This proves especially helpful when handling a call which is challenging for some reason. Mohammed is really encouraged by the results and decides to explore mindfulness further. He also becomes a strong advocate for it within his organisation.

Time out activity – if you are curious about how mindfulness might be useful within your work life, the following prompts should prove a useful starting point:

1. Choose an everyday work activity that you will carry out with mindful awareness for about a week.

2. Once you have chosen an activity, commit to focus intently on this whenever you carry it out, for one week. Before carrying out the activity, use a deep breath to bring yourself firmly into the present moment. Start the activity and try to focus only on this. Every time your attention wanders, gently guide it back to the activity.

3. Each time you carry out the activity, take a few moments to reflect on what happened. How did it feel? Were there any surprises or differences? What was the impact of really focusing all your attention on the activity?

4. Once the week is over, reflect on what the experience has taught you. Consider whether it has been helpful and whether you might want to continue or extend the practice.

Starting to bring a more mindful approach to work can help us step out of auto-pilot where we just react to stress and pressure, rather than choosing a response that is more likely to be helpful. If we can step out of auto-pilot, we may start to cultivate the ability to deal with life's challenges in a clear-minded, calm, healthy and assertive way.

Useful links and Resources

If you would like to explore mindfulness a little more, here are a few resources that are a good place to start:

Puddicombe, A. (2012). *Get Some Headspace: 10 minutes can make all the difference*. London: Hodder & Stoughton.

Alidina, S. (2014). *Mindfulness for Dummies*. Chichester: John Wiley & Sons.

The Headspace App available in the App Store.

See: www.mindful.org/meditation/mindfulness-getting-started/.

Shift Work

Most health-related call centres will run on a shift basis with most operating 24 hours a day, seven days a week. Staff will often need to work a range of shifts, including overnight. Some people are attracted to this type of work because of the shift pattern. For many, being able to work nights, evenings or weekends is beneficial because it helps with issues like childcare. However, shift work can sometimes have a negative impact on your social life and wellbeing. Here are some staff comments in relation to shift work:

'It's just the nature of the job.'

'It works around my personal commitments.'

'I prefer to do shift work.'

'I have no other option.'

'Flexible.'

'Fits around my other job.'

'Happened to fall into the job role and it was a requirement.'

It is clear that for some people, the advantages of shift work outweigh the disadvantages. However, there is research to support the fact that shift work can negatively impact on people's health. In one study, shift workers were more likely to report fair or bad general health (28% of men and women) than non-shift workers (21% of men and 23% of women).

Top tips for taking care of yourself before and during your night shift

Pre-night shift
- Physical exercise the evening before your night shift can help you get a good night's sleep.
- Stay up later than usual the night before your night shift. The aim of this is to sleep in the next morning to adjust your body clock slightly. Try and have a nap during the day before your night shift.

Day of the night shift
- The idea is to get some sleep, so try and do what's possible for you – get up late, sleep during the day or have a long nap before starting work.
- Eat well during the day and keep hydrated.
- Avoid too much exercise or other activities which could cause you to feel very tired during the night.
- Don't eat a very heavy meal before going on to your shift as this can make you tired.

The night shift
- Keep hydrated. A human adult is composed of roughly between 50–65% water, so it stands to reason that we need to keep hydrated. Call centres can often have dry atmospheres due to heating and air conditioning. You will often be doing a lot of talking over the course of a shift, so it is important to keep your mouth well hydrated.
- Eat well. Bring food from home rather than relying on sugary or fast foods which can cause an energy slump and might affect the care you give to callers.
- Avoid caffeine as this could affect sleep the next day.
- Take your allocated breaks.
- Do not drive if you realise you are too tired from your shift. This endangers your life and others.

Between night shifts
- Eat breakfast and avoid caffeine.
- Sleep once you have had breakfast. Do not skip sleep if you are working that night. The importance of sleep cannot be overestimated. Being well rested is essential for good emotional, mental and physical health. It is very hard to listen to people in need for long periods when you feel tired or jaded. Responding sensitively and empathetically is much easier when we feel physically and emotionally healthy. Sleep is essential in this respect. Critical thinking and effective decision making is significantly impacted when we do not get enough good-quality sleep, so make it a high priority.
- Try to avoid exposure to artificial lights when you are trying to sleep as they emit a blue light which research has shown interferes with sleep. This includes lights, screens, telephones, televisions, etc.
- Avoid committing to activities during the day. It is very important to recharge before your next shift as your role relies on clear thinking and being alert.
- Eat well and keep hydrated. Avoid alcohol during the day as this can severely interrupt sleep patterns. Additionally, you have no way of being sure that the alcohol will be out of your system by the time you start work.

Day off before going back onto day shifts
- Eat a good breakfast.
- Sleep for a shorter time in the day.
- Eat well and keep hydrated.
- Sleep at your usual time.

Summary

The role of call handler whilst rewarding, can be stressful and demanding. Your employer is obligated to take steps to protect the health and safety of staff, but you also have responsibilities. It is vitally important that you take active steps to look after your health and wellbeing at work to avoid 'burning out'. This includes looking after both your physical health, and your mental health and wellbeing. This chapter has included a number of factors that can help such as effective workstation hygiene and handwashing, developing an effective work-life balance, stress management, exercise and mindfulness, but there are many more strategies that you may personally find useful. Taking some time to identify what keeps you well and happy at work, and then committing to doing these regularly is important in order to develop healthy habits that stick.

References and Further Reading

Chartered Institute of Personnel Development (2016). *Growing the Health and Well-being Agenda: From First Steps to Full Potential*. Available at: https://www.cipd.co.uk/Images/health-well-being-agenda_2016-first-steps-full-potential_tcm18-10453.pdf (last accessed 8 June 2018).

Lyubomirsky, S. and Layous, K. (2013). How do simple positive activities increase well-being? *Current Directions in Psychological Science*, 22(1): 57–62.

Mind (2013). Work is biggest cause of stress in people's lives. Available at: https://www.mind.org.uk/news-campaigns/news/work-is-biggest-cause-of-stress-in-peoples-lives/#.WxpTDkgvyUk (last accessed: 20 June 2018).

NHS Choices (2018). *Your Health, Your Choices*. Available at: www.nhs.uk/Livewell/insomnia/Pages/bedtimeritual.aspx (last accessed 11 May 2017).

Pierce, H. and Lilly, M.M. (2012). Duty-related trauma exposure in 911 telecommunicators: considering the risk for posttraumatic stress. *Journal of Traumatic Stress*, 25(2): 211–215.

Querstret, D., Cropley, M. and Fife-Schaw, C. (2016). Internet-based instructor-led mindfulness for work-related rumination, fatigue, and sleep: assessing facets of mindfulness as mechanisms of change. A randomized waitlist control trial. *Journal of Occupational Health Psychology*, 22(2): 153–169.

Chapter 11: Professional Development

Learning Objectives

By the end of this chapter you will be able to:

- Recognise the importance of continuing professional development (CPD)
- Explain what CPD is and whose responsibility this is
- Summarise the contribution of reflective practice to CPD
- Describe the Gibbs model of reflection
- Explain the benefits of using a reflective journal
- State a range of approaches to learning different skills
- Describe other sources of learning that can contribute to CPD.

Introduction

Everyone working within the provision of healthcare has a responsibility to provide care which is safe, up to date and effective. A continued commitment to developing yourself professionally is important in this respect, because healthcare is a dynamic and evolving phenomenon. What was good practice ten years ago may not be best practice now because the knowledge and evidence base about what makes good healthcare is constantly developing. Anyone involved in healthcare has a responsibility to develop themselves 'professionally', not just registered professionals such as doctors and nurses.

What is Continuing Professional Development?

Continuing professional development (CPD) encompasses all of the activities that healthcare staff undertake, both formal and informal, to maintain, update, develop and enhance their professional skills, knowledge and attitudes. Your employer has a responsibility to help ensure you are adequately trained and developed for your role, but this does not remove your responsibility to focus on your own practice and potential areas for development.

Here are some key principles to bear in mind when considering your own CPD:

- Take proactive steps to identify what you need to learn and what areas for development you have. Use any tools at your disposal to identify learning needs such as call review activities and feedback from colleagues/patients.
- Regard development as a continuous part of everyday work, rather than a series of one-off events
- Regular investment in learning should be seen as an essential part of your professional life, not as an optional extra.
- The emphasis should be on learning from a wide range of activities. Become aware of your learning style but also be prepared to move out of your comfort zone. Remember that different types of learning need different skills.
- There should be an emphasis on outcomes – answering the questions 'What did you learn from this experience?' and 'How can you apply this learning?'
- Set yourself clear learning objectives that should serve your own goals and those of your organisation.

Reflective Practice as a Form of CPD

Training courses and qualifications can only go so far in supporting your development. Your effectiveness at work relies on learning by doing, from successes and mistakes. Your own experiences at work can be a source of powerful learning – but it requires thought and commitment to maximise this. Reflective practice, which is one of the most vital tools in the armoury of any lifelong learner, is an approach that links your thinking with your actions. Reflective practice is about examining your own actions to identify potential improvements and developments to your practice, with the ultimate aim of improving patient care. As a reflective learner, you should be able to use your experience as a positive source of learning even when things don't go as well as you would wish.

A Reflective Model

There are several models you can use to help focus your reflective practice. Popular models include Gibbs [1988], Johns [1995] and Rolfe et al. [2001]. Gibbs' reflective cycle is probably one of the most commonly used models in healthcare reflection and is outlined below. This is a simple-to-follow model that invites you to look back on an experience and then consider the different

elements in specific stages [Gibbs, 1988]. Let's consider these stages in a little more detail

Description

This should provide a brief overview of what happened, trying just to focus on the facts. Cover the incident from start to finish, but do not spend time describing things that were not significant.

Feelings

Recall and explore the things that were going through your mind:

- How were you feeling when the event started?
- What were you thinking about at the time?
- How did it make you feel?

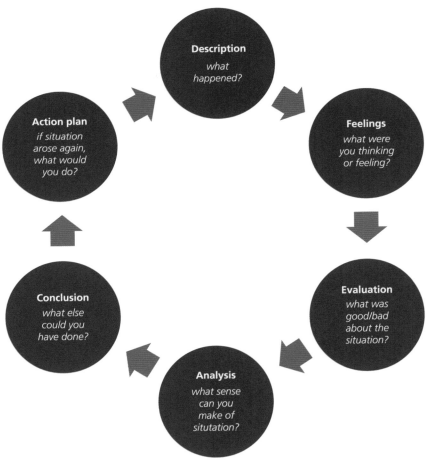

Figure 11.1 Gibbs' reflective model
Source: Gibbs (1988)

- What did other people's actions/words make you think?
- How did you feel about the outcome?
- What do you think about it now?

Evaluation

Evaluation gives you the opportunity to consider what went well and what did not go so well in any experience. This may be based on your own actions or the actions of others. Your reflections here should try to balance positives and negatives. You should be searching for experiences you would repeat in the future and also experiences where – given the opportunity again – you would do things differently.

Analysis

Analysis should form the largest part of any reflection. In this part of the cycle, you get to explore all of the issues that you have highlighted as part of your description, feelings and evaluation. You should now consider these points one at a time and review what made them either particularly positive or an area for development. You may also want to compare the experience to previous similar situations and consider what was unique about that particular experience that impacted on your performance.

Questions you could ask yourself are:

- Why did I take that decision or make certain choices and what impact did it have?
- What was influencing my thinking or decision making at the time?
- How would I do it differently in the future?

Conclusion

Now you have successfully dissected the incident, you need to make sense of it. This might include drawing conclusions about your own and other people's behaviour in terms of how they contributed to the event.

Action Plan

Now you have drawn some conclusions, you are in a position to plan for next time. This is about getting clear on what you would like to do as a result of this incident and what you've learnt. It may help to consider the following:

- How will you do it?
- When will you do it?

- Where will you do it?
- Who will be part of the action?

Keeping a Reflective Journal

You may want to consider maintaining a reflective journal whilst working as a call handler. This can be a really useful way of analysing the care you provide, highlighting your strengths, identifying areas for development and tracking improvements. Having a 'system' for reflection is useful. Everyone reflects on a near-constant basis throughout their life, but lending some structure to this process can make it a powerful tool for learning and developing.

Please provide details of the event/situation – call taken/feedback/other areas of your work

This event/situation can be positive or negative.

Description

I took a call and spoke to a caller whose friend had collapsed and stopped breathing.

I struggled with the call and a colleague had to intervene and take over.

Feelings

I felt really anxious and panicky because it was the first time I'd dealt with someone in this state. I felt embarrassed that someone had to take over. I felt a certain amount of resentment that I wasn't fully prepared. I was relieved she got the care she needed, but it has made me nervous about my ability to do this job.

Evaluation

Nothing about the call went well! Apart from perhaps the fact that I was able to get help from a colleague quickly. I didn't use the system correctly and didn't know how to correct my mistake.

Analysis

I decided to get help because I could tell this was an extremely urgent situation. I think the panic in the caller's voice got my adrenaline going on overdrive. On reflection, I know that I do know what to do, but I panicked and a sort of mist came over me making it hard for me to think straight. I think my feelings of resentment were actually a bit defensive – I should have been able to handle the call but I couldn't. I must recognise that it's still early days for me in this job, and, looking at things positively, I did get help really quickly because I recognised that time mattered.

Conclusion

Because this was the first time I'd handled such a call, my nerves and the caller's anxiety got the better of me. I need to make sure I have some techniques for calming myself and the caller down if this sort of thing happens again. I also need to practice dealing with some more really serious calls so that I am more prepared. And I also need to keep reminding myself how to backtrack if I make a mistake.

Action Plan

1. I'm going to dig out some of my training materials and ask a colleague to role play some emergency calls with me. I can also make some deliberate mistakes navigating my way through the system and see how quickly I can backtrack to where I need to be. I'll speak to my team leader tomorrow about when this can happen, but will stress it as a priority.

2. I'm also going to do some reading tonight about how to manage high emotion during a call. We covered this in training, but it will mean more now, after this experience.

3. My friend talked about mindfulness and how this can help in stressful situations. I think I'll give her a ring at the weekend to find out more.

Remember that reflection is not just about focusing on mistakes or things that did not go as well as you would have liked. Identifying what went well is equally important; it is a way to reinforcing this in future practice.

Whilst a reflective journal is a powerful developmental tool, it is possible to reflect and learn without writing things down, so don't let the impression that reflecting on practice must be a written process deter you! Sometimes, just talking an incident through with a colleague, using a structured process, can be just as powerful.

Different Learning Approaches

As an adult you are already a very accomplished learner, but you may not have thought very

much about your own personal approach to learning. Have a go at the following activity to get you thinking about how we learn different skills.

Time out activity – different ways of learning

Consider how you learned to do each of the activities below. If you have not already learned to do them, think about the methods that you would try to learn to do them now:

- Ride a bike?
- Drive a car?
- Speak a new language?
- Bake bread?
- Be a partner (business or personal)?

Chances are you listed a range of different teaching and learning approaches, because different skills require different methods.

Learning to ride a bike can involve a number of different tactics including trial and error, getting someone to steady the bike and finding a safe place to make mistakes. It often involves moving outside of one's comfort zone. Some people cannot remember how they learned to ride a bike and think that it just came naturally. This is not uncommon – often once we've mastered a certain skill we cannot remember how we acquired it. Most drivers can, however, remember learning to drive a car. This can be a difficult process until the process of coordination becomes unconscious. Some people read a book to help them learn to drive, many take formal courses but this is often supplemented with practice in a relative's car. Most people need to learn the Highway Code but many road signs are learned through being a passenger in a car.

Learning a new language can involve classes, books, videos or by spending time in the relevant country. Baking bread, like driving a car, is not easy to learn from books or pictures as it involves a number of judgements (for instance about the consistency of the dough). An expert may be able to teach you a lot about this skill.

Learning to be a partner involves linking a range of skills and understanding. It involves interpersonal relationships and interactions that will change as circumstances change.

It involves learning about yourself as well as others. Here most people learn from experience, but some people may choose to supplement this by reading books about successful relationships.

It is clear that different skills need different teaching and learning methods. Some skills absolutely have to be practised, such as riding a bike, whereas others could be gained from reading, such as learning a foreign vocabulary. Other skills are so complex that they might take a range of different approaches (such as learning to drive a car). Passing your driving test will usually have involved observation, practice, learning the Highway Code and inevitably, reflecting and learning from a few mistakes along the way.

The skills and competencies you need for your role will also require different approaches to learning (e.g. the symptoms of certain medical conditions could potentially be learned just from personal reading and research). Learning how best to demonstrate empathy and warmth to a caller in distress might potentially be learned through a combination of approaches such as observation of a colleague, reading about the underpinning theory, having a go either with a real caller or within a role play, feedback from someone else and personal reflection. Challenging your own personal stereotypes and biases might best be learned through a process of completing case studies and group discussion.

In thinking about your professional development it is important to consider the best way(s) of learning the particular skill.

Time out activity – sources of learning

Before reading on, spend a few minutes thinking about all the potential sources of learning available to you in your role as a call handler.

Summary

Your workplace is a rich source of learning that probably provides a mix of formal and informal development opportunities. These may include:

- Coaching and mentoring (both receiving and providing can be rich sources of learning).
- Call review – reviewing your own calls, having a peer review them or having a supervisor review them.
- Feedback – for example, from a peer, supervisor, patient or other professional colleague.
- Personal research and reading.
- Attendance-based workshops and courses.
- E-learning and other distance learning courses.
- Academic study.
- Reflection.
- Discussion and debate.
- Case studies.
- Role play.
- Observation of colleagues.
- Shadowing to find out about others' roles.
- Secondments.
- Visits to other organisations.
- Attending forums, seminars, special interest groups and conferences.

References and Further Reading

Gibbs, G. (1988). *Learning by Doing: A Guide to Teaching and Learning Methods*. Further Education Unit. Oxford: Oxford Polytechnic. Available at: https://www.brookes.ac.uk/students/upgrade/study-skills/reflective-writing-gibbs/.

Johns, C. (1995). Framing learning through reflection within Carper's fundamental ways of knowing in nursing. *Journal of Advanced Nursing* (22)2: 226–234

Rolfe, G., Freshwater, D., Jasper, M. (2001). *Critical reflection in nursing and the helping professions: a user's guide*. Basingstoke: Palgrave Macmillan.

Index